A PLUME BOOK

THE SWOLY BIBLE

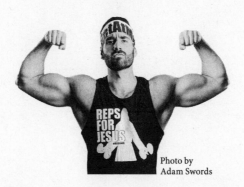

Photo by
Adam Swords

A self-proclaimed expert on everything, **Dom Mazzetti** is an Italian American bro in his early twenties who hails from the tristate area. Confidently stupid but with good intentions, Dom refuses to grow up and takes glee in his day-to-day, responsibility-free existence. At his core—way down deep to his perfectly sculpted core—Dom is a great guy, just misunderstood. Dom is the type of guy who will give you the shirt off his back, even if you don't want his shirt, just so he can be shirtless. This is his first book.

DOM MAZZETTI

THE SWOLY BIBLE

THE BRO SCIENCE
WAY OF LIFE

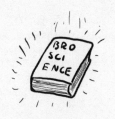

A PLUME BOOK

PLUME
An imprint of Penguin Random House LLC
375 Hudson Street
New York, New York 10014

P Plume is a registered trademark and its colophon is a trademark
of Penguin Random House LLC

LIBRARY OF CONGRESS CATALOGING-IN-PUBLICATION DATA
has been applied for.

Printed in the United States of America
10 9 8 7 6 5 4 3 2 1

PUBLISHER'S NOTE: This is a work of satire. Neither the publisher nor the author is engaged
in rendering professional advice or services to the individual reader, nor shall the publisher or
author be liable or responsible for any loss or damage allegedly arising from any information
in this book.

Dedicated to Mike & Gian

CONTENTS

Introduction   xi

Muscle Glossary   xiv

What Is Bro Science?   xix

The Seven Stages of the Evolution of the Lifting Man   xxiii

Stage 1: Primordial Ooze

Chapter 1: Life Before Lifting   3

Stage 2: Tadpole

Chapter 2: The Brofessor   9

Chapter 3: What Is a Pump?   12

Chapter 4: Rookie Mistakes   15

Chapter 5: Locker Room Etiquette   21

Chapter 6: Should I Take Pre-Workout?   25

Chapter 7: You May Now Approach the Bench   29

Chapter 8: How to Deadlift   32

Chapter 9: Dumbbell (Dombell) Curls   38

Chapter 10: Don't Be a Half Repper   42

Chapter 11: Yo, Can I Get a Spot?   46

Chapter 12: Whey Too Much Brotein   50

Stage 3: Brotégé

Chapter 13: How to Find a Gym Buddy   55

Chapter 14: How to Take a Selfie   60

Chapter 15: How to Hit on a Girl in the Gym   65

Chapter 16: What Type of Fitness Chick Are You?   70

Chapter 17: One-Night Stands   77

Chapter 18: How to Pack for Music Festivals   83

Chapter 19: Beach Weekend Pump Workout   88

Chapter 20: How to Take Your Shirt Off   92

Chapter 21: Gym Buddy Problems   96

Chapter 22: There Will Be Grunts   100

Chapter 23: Look Big, Get Big   104

Chapter 24: What Your Gym Gear Says About You   108

Stage 4: Gym Bro

Chapter 25: How to Skip Leg Day   115

Chapter 26: What Is CrossFit?   119

Chapter 27: How to Get Your Girlfriend to Start Lifting   122

Chapter 28: Fitness Tips for Basic Chicks   126

Chapter 29: Diets   129

Chapter 30: How to Eat Chicken Without Wanting to
Kill Yourself   132

Chapter 31: What Is IIFYM?   139

Chapter 32: How to Bulk   142

Chapter 33: How to Cut   145

Chapter 34: Spring Break   149

Stage 5: Gym Rat

Chapter 35: New Gym Checklist   157

Chapter 36: How to Get Hyped for a Lift   160

Chapter 37: Why Rest Days Are Bullshit   166

Chapter 38: Extreme Pump Secrets—Home Edition   170

Chapter 39: How to Fix Injuries and Imbalances   174

Chapter 40: How to Be Alpha All the Time   177

Chapter 41: Most Alpha Chest Exercises   182

Chapter 42: Most Alpha Back Exercises   185

Chapter 43: Least Alpha Exercises   188

Chapter 44: How to Defeat Your Gym Nemesis   192

Chapter 45: Do You Even Lift?   196

Stage 6: Monster

Chapter 46: Pros and Cons of Taking Steroids   199

Chapter 47: People You Hate at the Gym   205

Chapter 48: How to Declare War on New Year's
Resolutioners   210

Chapter 49: How to Bring a Beginner to the Gym   213

Chapter 50: Meathead Goals   218

Stage 7: Freak Beast

Conclusion   225

Bronus   227

Acknowledgments   229

INTRODUCTION

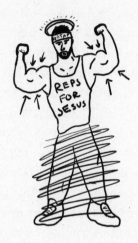

Yo. The name is Dom Mazzetti and I'm the founder of Bro Science Life.

Now, before I get into what exactly Bro Science is, let me tell you a little bit about myself.

Like many of our world's leaders, I hail from the great state of New Jersey.

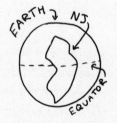

I'm not talking about the New Jersey you're familiar with from the TV show *Jersey Shore*, though I did definitely tear up Seaside every weekend during high school. No, I grew up in small-farm-town Jersey. No lie, kids would drive their fucking tractors to school. In my town, you had to create your entertainment or else you'd be sittin' on your ass all weekend. We'd throw bonfire parties in our neighbor's backyard while they were on vacation. Caused a few forest fires, but no one needs to know that. But even as a young buck, I knew if I didn't get the hell out of New Jersey eventually, I was destined to become another townie who takes week-end trips to Hoboken. The thing about New Jersey is that when you are in it, your only goal is to get the fuck out, and once you do get out, it becomes your biggest pride. Kind of like prison. And I knew that a scrawny dude from the 'burbs ain't gonna fare well in prison.

My only choice was to pull an El Chapo and start my own life. Today, many of you know me as a ripped muscle god who basically started the Internet, but that wasn't always the case. I have a secret I'm finally ready to share with you. Hold on . . . I am getting a little choked up . . . this never happens . . . a shot of tequila for courage . . . okay, here it goes: I, Dom Mazzetti, used to be small. What a pussy, I know.

You never notice how small you are until you're standing next to someone bigger than you. Eventually, I just started noticing people becoming bigger than me and the larger they got, the better they got.

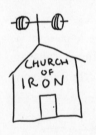

Now, I ain't no mathematician, but it's clear as day that to be alpha is to be huge. $E = mc^{Huge}$. I needed to get there. I needed to not feel like a complete squeeb around chicks or always wonder, "What if you were jacked, Dom?" Fuck that. I needed to do something. And I wasn't about to volunteer for random drug testing by playing a sport, so I did the next best thing: I hit the gym, aka the Church of Iron. My complete personal transformation into what you see today is all because of the gym.

Getting huge is all I know and it is my duty to share with you all that I have learned.

I will never forget the day I was introduced to the gym. It all started because this chick I asked on a date sophomore year of high school turned me down and proceeded to get drilled out by some yoked-out very cool community college bro. How could I hate on that guy?

He had everything: a sick Mitsubishi Lancer with a spoiler, the hottest chick in my grade, and a tattoo of a baseball on his back. But even without all that, the guy had gains. See, what I came to realize about getting jacked is if you take everything else away, you're still jacked. Having mass is all you need. That very day, I walked into the school gym and aimlessly moved weight around until a random 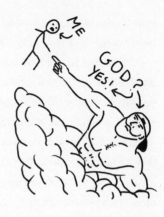 bro asked me to spot him. This moment changed my life because this "random bro" was not random. He was in fact sent to me from a higher power. He was my muscle angel, aka my brofessor.

From that day forth I was hitting the gym so much that I eventually started a YouTube channel dedicated to the craft called Bro Science Life. Bro Science Life chronicles all I have learned and continue to learn in the gym, and now, at the request of bros everywhere, I present to you my findings in book form. *The Swoly Bible* is a field manual on all things Bro Science. For example, let's say a snowstorm hits your town and your gym is closed, but you took a rest day yesterday and now you're small. What do you do?

BRO TIP: You crack open *The Swoly Bible* and skip right to Chapter 38: Extreme Pump Secrets—Home Edition.

Now, you may be wondering what "swoly" means. "Swoly" is derived from the Latin, "swollen," which in French is "swole," which in English is "big." To be swole is the single greatest accomplishment of your life, and lucky for you, you can be swole at least once a day if you follow my guidance. *The Swoly Bible* is here to learn you on all the ways of acquiring swole, how to maintain that swole, and most important, how to transport that heavy cargo, aka your body, outside the gym and into the real world.

Welcome to the first and last book you will ever need to read. *The Swoly Bible* is meant to become a part of you. A text you will carry with you and consult during hard times and good. *The Swoly Bible* is not fiction. It is science. Bro Science.

Now, before you read any further, it is important that you know your way around *The Swoly Bible* just like you would want to know your way around a gym before setting foot in one. Get familiar with the muscle glossary below before getting your brain swole on.

MUSCLE GLOSSARY

Alpha: The top dog. The perception of being the biggest, strongest dude in a given area or situation.

ATP: Adenosine triphosphate, the source of energy in your body that keeps you going.

Body Dysmorphia: When you look in the mirror and think you are smaller than you are. This is the biggest and the worst problem of all time.

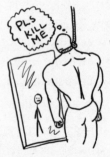

Branch Chain Amino Acids (BCAAs): A powder you drink to increase muscle growth over time. They give you consistent energy, rather than an all-at-once burst like pre-workout does. The main three amino acids in BCAAs are leucine, isoleucine, and valine. You can typically see meatheads carrying around gallon jugs full of BCAAs.

Brofessor: The individual who brought you into the gym and bestowed upon you the knowledge of Bro Science. *See also* The Swoly Spirit.

Brotégé: You.

Bumper Plates: Plates made of solid rubber. Typically used in CrossFit.

Church: The gym.

CrossFit: A recent fitness trend involving a bunch of sheep jumping around in a room and passing it off as actual fitness.

Cutoff: Any shirt that once had sleeves but no longer does. Aka, a real shirt.

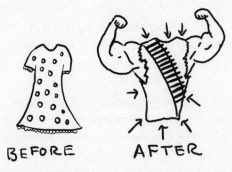

BEFORE   AFTER

Dropset: Immediately following up one exercise with the same exact exercise but with less weight.

Free Weights: Weight that is not attached to anything, like a cable or a machine. A free weight is a weight you can grab and lift and take anywhere with you. I carry two 35lb dumbbells with me everywhere I go. Despite the name, free weights aren't actually free, so don't try to remove them from their sacred shrines.

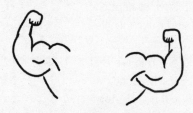

Gnar Pump: The best pre-workout in the game, made by yours truly.

Invisible Lat Syndrome: When you work out so much that you think your lats are so fucking huge that they won't allow your arms to fall at your side.

Latissimi Dorsi, aka Lats: The muscles on your back that make you get that sick V taper.

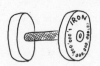

Lifting: If you need to look this up, we have a lot of work to do. Lifting means to lift weights. To say "Fuck you" to gravity, I'm moving this shit because I can.

Machines: Anything that you see in a gym that isn't a free weight is a machine. Machines work well for certain exercises, but can be restricting. Free your muscles by lifting free weights.

Macros: Macronutrients that make up food: protein, carbs, and fat. Measured in grams (g). Essential for survival, aka growth.

'Mirin': The act of admiring someone, or yourself. Usually yourself.

Personal Record (PR): When you set a new personal lift record. For example, you just hit a new PR of 215lbs on bench and haven't stopped talking about it.

Plateau: Stages in your lifting career when it gets difficult to lift more weight past a certain point.

Pre-Workout: A workout supplement that you take before you lift. A form of powdered lightning and strength chemicals that gives you the power of Zeus.

Pump: A pump is what happens when you lift and your muscles fill with blood and magic and become bigger. A pump is like that primo street smack that gets everyone hooked and coming back for more, forever. But, like all great things in life, a pump never lasts forever.

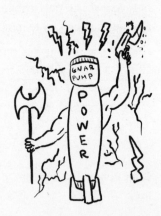

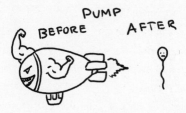

Reps: The number of times you repeat a specific exercise in one set. Like, "I did a million reps of curls for four sets yesterday."

Sets: The number of times you do an exercise. Like, "I did four sets of curls yesterday."

Shaker Cup: A plastic cup that you put various muscle powders into, shake, and drink from. It's like an adult sippy cup.

Split: How one splits up his/her workout routines.

Superset (pronounced *supa set*): Immediately following up one exercise with a different one.

Tank: A piece of clothing with no sleeves, exposing chest and back. The greatest item of fashion to ever be created.

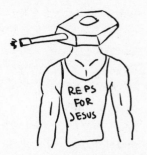

Tech: Futuristic gym clothing and accessories that make you look and feel like a space-age muscle warrior, but which are generally useless.

Test: Testosterone. Test makes you a man. It can be manufactured in your body by working out like a beast. It can also be injected into your body because you are a fuckin' beast.

Congratulations, you are now armed with the brain gains necessary to achieve actual gains. Mass is officially in session.

WHAT IS BRO SCIENCE?

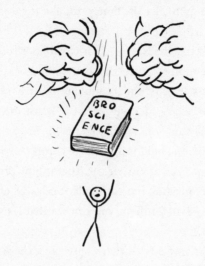

What's bigger than science? BRO SCIENCE. Bro Science is fucking huge. It is like if science took steroids. Except you don't have to go to college to become a Bro Scientist. Your education can be gotten in any gym around the world. In these gyms you will encounter Bro Scientists of all types. See, in its purest form, Bro Science is lifting advice that comes from a bro who looks like he works out more than you do. His size means he's lifted more weight than you, has hooked up with more chicks, and is overall better at life.

Every jacked guy in the gym is a gold mine full of unfounded tips on how to get big. When you first start hitting the gym, you might feel nervous about approaching a muscle god and asking him questions about his workout. But don't worry, young grasshopper: You are already way ahead of the game just by opening *The Swoly Bible*. In fact, you are being learned by the biggest Bro Scientist in the game. You're welcome. But the fact of the matter is, even I, Dom Mazzetti, can't know everything there is to know about lifting because I will never be as big as I can be. Bro Science is an ever-evolving field. The more time you spend in the gym, aka the boneyard, aka the dungeon, the more Bro Science you will learn.

Bro Science is like the Native American folklore of the gym, passed down from generation to generation of gym buddies. It is ancient wisdom from the muscle gods, and it should be taken as sacred advice. For example, my bro, who's fucking JACKED (trust me, you should see him; HMU if you want some pix), told me his Bro Science, then I told my bro, and he's gonna tell his bro, aka his brotégé, which in French is protégé, which is a type of muscle car. That is how Bro Science works. You don't need to question the knowledge bestowed upon you because every time you look in a mirror you can see that it's working. It's not that complicated.

Now, just like any advice that's based in experience rather than actual fact, there's good advice and there's bad advice. Here are some examples of good Bro Science:

Hitting skull crushers on a decline gets you a better stretch in your triceps. Ipso facto, get big.

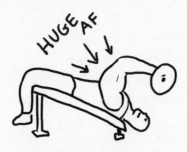

Jump rope between sets. Keeps your heart rate up and gets your calves big. Trust me, I just watched *The Fighter*.

Here are some examples of bad Bro Science:

Spinning the weights when you bench because you think it gets you bigger faster because of gravity.

No. Look around, everyone's posting your stupidity to their Snapchat stories.

Don't do squats—they're bad for your knees.

You're a pussy.

Bro Science is great, because you don't have to waste time explaining real science. The proof is literally standing in front of you, and there's no way you're not looking right at it because the proof is fucking huge. As long as the dude dishing out Bro Science is bigger than you, there's nothing you can say to him. Just get learned. No matter what stage in the lifting evolution you are in, there will always be another bro who is more qualified (bigger) than you. I don't need science. My eyes just proved it. Bro Science: 50 percent magic, 50 percent fact, 100 percent results.

Now, do you want to major in regular science, *or* would you rather skip school altogether, stop traffic, and give yourself an honorary doctorate in the most important field known to man? That's what I thought.

The Greats of Bro Science

Arnold Schwarzenegger	Zeus
Mahatma Gaindhi	Bisaac Newton
Swolbroham Lincoln	Ronnie Coleman
Malcom Flex	Barzan, King of the Gainforest

Gnarles Barwin

Rawnald Reagan

Biclops

Broseidon

Neil "The Mass" Trison

BarBar Binks

PRD2

Dumbbelldore

Bulkahontas

6Pac Shacore

Bob Gnarley

Walter Weight aka Bisenberg

Bill Plates

Strong F. Kennedy

THE SEVEN STAGES OF THE EVOLUTION OF THE LIFTING MAN

Most humans walking the earth today came into existence through the normal stages of evolution, which is super boring. Those muscle beasts you see in the gym? They blasted through normal evolution and underwent the seven stages of the lifting man. Normal humans evolved from apes, but guys like me, we evolved into apes. Yeah, that's right. Suck it, Darwin. Each stage of *The Swoly Bible* is divided up according to the seven stages of the evolution of the lifting man. You need to know which category you currently fall under so you know your past, present, and future. And I will tell you one thing, the future ain't always pretty, but it is fucking huge.

Stage 1. Primordial Ooze: You exist, and that is about it.

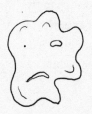

Stage 2. Tadpole: Your evolution begins here, because this is where your gains begin.

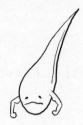

Stage 3. Brotégé: Approximately six months after you start lifting and you finally have a hint of muscle. You are at the height of your confidence, because body dysmorphia has not kicked in yet.

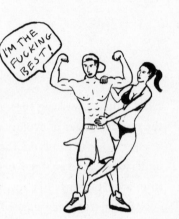

Stage 4. Gym Bro: You have some experience and knowledge under your belt. You have a solid gym regimen and can even spit a little Bro Science to the younguns. People definitely can tell you lift by now. You dumped your girlfriend because she is not as pretty as you.

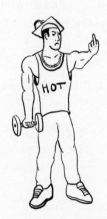

Stage 5. Gym Rat: You are scientifically considered to be jacked. You have conquered consistently getting laid, but you are now only interested in being the biggest guy in the gym.

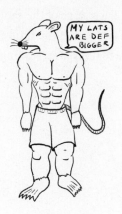

Stage 6. Monster: You are huge and have full-blown image issues. People think you are scary and that makes you happy. You may or may not have experimented with steroids.

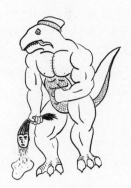

Stage 7. Freak Beast: You exist solely to be big and have grown a hooved foot.

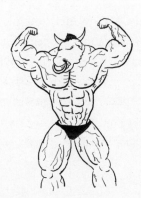

Each stage of the evolution should excite you more and more. I've laid out your entire future step-by-step in *The Swoly Bible*. Now all you have to do is keep reading.

STAGE 1

Primordial Ooze

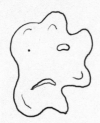

Welcome to existence. You are officially a form of life. Now, before you go and start celebrating, remember that you are nothing. You are incomplete matter that does not matter. You are the extra sperm that did not make it. No, never mind, you are the sperm that got spit out. You are gross and undeveloped. You are a weird soupy conglomeration of molecules that cannot lift anything, because the Primordial Ooze stage is the period before you start lifting, commonly referred to as BL. Yeah, you physically exist, but you are making zero impact on the universe right now. If you remain in the ooze state, you may be technically alive, but it is like living your entire life in a coma. Keep reading to find out if you are ooze.

CHAPTER 1

Life Before Lifting

Honestly, I am not even sure what there is to say about life before lifting weights. All I know is that there was no science, no text, no research or literature dating back to the time period BL. Because of scientific advancements, we now know that life existed Before Lifting, but there is nothing worth talking about. Man was a barnacle on society, a fucking troglodyte, before he started moving mass. Nothing mattered until man grew a pair of arms, swam to the surface from miles beneath the sea, and climbed his ass onto land. It was in that moment, my friend, that life truly began.

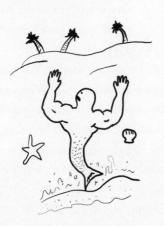

Now, if you haven't yet lifted, you are still in the ooze state. To be human means that you have to be in a solid state, and you are far from there at this point. The fact is, you have not been to church yet, and you have not met the Swoly Spirit.

It's important that you recognize where you came from. I know where you came from, but I ain't your dad. You can call me Daddy, though. Your mom already does. Ouch. But let's take a deeper look at who you are at this point in time. You are young, but not the cool kind of young like Young Jeezy. By definition, "young" means that you have not grown. It does not matter how old you are because the fact is that you have not started lifting yet, which means that you have not grown, ipso facto, you are young.

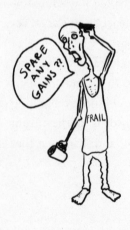

And you are definitely scrawny. Being scrawny is worse than being skinny, and that is really tough to do. Being scrawny goes beyond what you look like—scrawny engulfs your personality. When you are scrawny, even your soul is frail and weak. People pity you and want to give you their leftover Chili's. The only positive to being scrawny is that you can literally lift any weight and it will add muscle to your body. Anyway, I am not trying to ruin your confidence 30 pages into this book.

Just kidding, you have no confidence. You are like the fat kid from *Rocket Power*, but at least he had friends. When a human owns a sense of confidence, that human is able to lift weight. The more weight one can lift, the more confident one is. I can lift more fucking weight than Atlas, and that homie had the world on his shoulders. I have a better shoulder cap than him, too. Plus, Earth is not even heavy. I do core exercises with Jupiter.

At the end of the day, you are aware that you cannot keep living in the ooze state because ooze is not a state. New Jersey, Virginia, Miami . . . now, those are states. You are like my best friend, Boosh: You do not have any options, you are not very talented, and your personality is marginal at best. You simply will not be able to navigate the world (i.e., the gym) as primordial ooze.

Sorry not sorry if my words come off as harsh, but the fact is that if you want to be somebody you only have one option: gym. This is that moment when you make the decision to evolve, to become something, to wake the fuck up and be alive. This is the moment you decide to start lifting. You want to lift for the sole purpose of looking good, getting girls, and fixing that horrible genetic dice roll you ended up with. So tee up a Facebook event and invite your 89 friends, because you are about to have your *Bar* Mitzvah. There is no turning back now, in your life and in this book. If you turn one page back both will blow up. Good luck.

STAGE 2

Tadpole

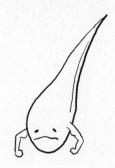

Ever wonder why arms are the most important part of your body? Because they were the first to develop, physiologically speaking. Not your brain, not your heart, and certainly not your legs. If the tadpole did not have arms, it would not have been able to climb ashore and invent the bench press. Take a moment to thank your muscle cannons and appreciate where you came from. Welcome to the Tadpole stage.

CHAPTER 2

The Brofessor

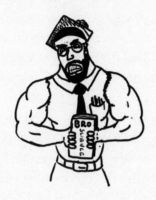

The Tadpole stage of evolution is a pivotal moment, but more important is how and why you started lifting in the first place. That honor belongs to your brofessor. Your brofessor is the most important person in your life. He's someone you can confide in and trust, for, like, two hours at a time three or four days every week. Your brofessor is the living and breathing inspiration right in front of you. He is proof that greatness is possible.

You may never truly understand why your first brofessor chose to learn you. Maybe your older sister overheard you saying how much you wanted to "get ripped" and forced her husband to lug your skeleton into the gym. Or maybe your college roommate saw you for the first time and didn't want to live with a pussy, so he convinced you to go to the boneyard after Comp 101. Some gym noobs find their brofessor on their own terms; others are lucky to have a brofessor assigned to them. However you end up in a gym, one fact is indisputable: No one ever starts going to the gym by themselves. That is like showing up to a party alone. You are going to stare at your phone for ten minutes then leave because everyone knows you're a virgin. So just be grateful that this bro entered your sad and pathetic life.

Once you have been introduced to the gym like some Freemason's initiation, you will begin copying everything your brofessor does. This is where you will start forming your personal foundation of Bro Science beliefs. You are like a sponge soaking up any fitness knowledge your brofessor leaks onto the gym floor. Your brofessor introduced you to this world; everything he says you take as fact because he created this world for you.

I met my brofessor in high school when he was hanging out in the parking lot drinking a shaker cup full of whey protein. This dude was fucking jacked. I asked him what was in the futuristic cup and he handed it to me. Tasted like chunky chocolate sap. I asked him why the hell he was drinking that stuff, and his only reply was, "Helps me recover." Recover from what? I needed to know. I started lightly stalking him and copying what he did in the gym until one day he came up to me and told me that if I kept deadlifting like that I was going to throw my back out before I was eighteen. From that day forward, I listened to everything he told me.

You must accept your brofessor as your spiritual guide and believe everything he says to you. If he tells you to tuck your shoulders back while benching, you tuck your fucking shoulders back. If your brofessor tells you that doing high reps makes your muscles more cut, you will believe this, no questions asked. Now, since you are susceptible to believing any knowledge, good or bad, that your brofessor feeds you, you better pray to the goddamn stars that you are blessed with a good brofessor. Ending up with a shitty brofessor is like having racist parents. No kid is born racist, but after years of hearing his parents' ignorance, he will grow up to be that kid who never left his hometown and thinks the Holocaust was made up by Hollywood Jews. Trust me: You do not want to get stuck in a conversation with this guy at the gym. And if you are this guy, it is too late because you will never realize the mental rapist that you have become. You are wasting my time and energy by the sheer force of your stupidity. In summary, a good brofessor is more important than good parents.

Assuming you have a decent brofessor, flash forward three months and you will have made some beginner gains that no one cares about or notices, except for you. Mirrors and reflective objects are slowly becoming your best friend because you are your best friend, because you are the best thing around.

Rules of Lifting with Your Brofessor

Never interrupt when he is speaking.

Always do what he is doing, even if you know it's wrong, which it isn't.

If he decides not to show up without telling you, don't question him.

If he tells you that you have more reps in you, listen to him. He knows you better than you know yourself, even if you just met yesterday.

Drink any liquid that he tells you to drink.

CHAPTER 3

What Is a Pump?

As if your brofessor has not taught you enough, he also introduced you to the most important achievement of your life: your first pump. Your first pump is a life-altering moment, but the loss of your first pump is even more important. It's an alpha and omega moment. A pump is when you witness actual change happen to your body as a result of lifting, only to see that change disappear a few hours later. You experienced what you could be and what you once were all in one day. It's a vicious cycle, but a necessary one.

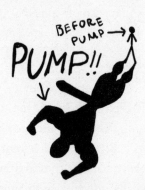

There is no way to describe a pump to someone who has never had a pump. It is like describing to Helen Keller how 3-D glasses work. She has never even seen a 3-D movie; she died before 3-D was invented. But that's what I'm here for: to do the impossible, so here goes.

By the standard definition, a pump is what happens when you are lifting and blood rushes to your muscles, swells them up, and makes them rock hard. But alas, young virgins, a pump is so much more than standard definition. When you get a pump, you are becoming the absolute biggest and best version of yourself for, like, two hours. A pump is instant gratification. It is the only thing in life that lets you know what you are doing is working. Think about it: When I am reading, I don't see my brain getting all huge and hard. Take that, school!

A pump is seeing your future. Once you see yourself with a pump you want to be that big all the time. Then once you get that big, your pump gets even bigger. No matter how hard you try you will never be as big as your pump. A pump is like tomorrow, and you can never reach tomorrow because once it is tomorrow, it is today again. But you will never stop chasing tomorrow because you always want to live another day and tomorrow never dies. What? What the fuck just happened? What did I just type? I blacked out. I think I came a little, too. What was I saying?

Okay, so if you are confused by everything I just said a pump was, let me simplify for you and myself with this list.

A pump is a boner for your entire body.

A pump is finishing third but getting the gold medal.

A pump is an impossible chase. You are Captain Ahab and your pump is your Moby Dick, and your dick is your dick.

A pump is achieving muscular arousal from your own reflection.

A pump is hitting that mushroom in Super Mario and growing two sizes, but you know that shit is going to leave before you can get to the boss, aka the club.

A pump is seeing God's dick, and then realizing it is yours.

A pump is like driving a Lamborghini into Cleopatra's butt.

A pump is getting cream-pied by God.

A pump is like riding a horse made out of dragons.

A pump is punching Jupiter with your dick and eating out the sun. There is nothing harder and there is nothing hotter.

A pump is a lot like hitting the snooze button. It feels great dreaming for five more minutes, but at some point you have to wake up.

A pump is seeing that one bicep vein under the right lighting, then telling people you compete.

A pump is typing the word "lie" then hitting bold and sending.

A pump is letting Jesus take the wheel while you rub one out and play Game Boy. Reps for Jesus.

A pump is that always DTF chick that will give you some butt reps, but will never let you cuddle.

A pump is getting a hug from your muscles.

A pump is like giving birth to a son and knowing he is going to be good at sports.

A pump is driving two jet skis at once, but one jet ski is a rhino farting lightning and the second jet ski is two jet skis.

A pump is the theory of evolution proven in an hour and a half.

A pump is clicking on related videos while watching porn. Once you go down that rabbit hole, you will never be satisfied with real life again.

A pump is more addictive than *Breaking Bad* and actual meth. But I am addicted to all three; call me Walter Weight.

A pump is like winning the blood lottery, but it is a scratch-off and you won just enough for tomorrow's ticket.

—◁▯——▯▷—

So welcome to the club, buddy. You will never be the same again, because the day you started lifting was the day you became forever small.

CHAPTER 4

Rookie Mistakes

The day you have been dreading has finally arrived: You have to go to the gym without your brofessor. He took eleven too many car bombs at the bar last night and still isn't awake. Respect. Now you are faced with a decision: Skip your workout today and lose all your gains, or reach into your pants, grab your nutsack, and drag yourself to the gym by it.

You still may have the crippling fear of being ridiculed since you are fairly new to the gym, but in reality nobody cares, because once again, you are small. No one is even looking at you, because you are not even big enough to see. It is, however, easy to spot your insecurity through the double XL hoodie draped over your nonexistent traps. But even though you are about as noticeable as the rack of dumbbells below 15lbs, you still do not want to brand yourself as a rookie. Here are some things to avoid.

Half Repping

Half repping is one of the most flagrant offenses in the gym. It is the act of not completing the full range of motion required to count as one whole repetition—in other words, you are putting in half the work. It means you are not interested in follow-through, hard work, and results.

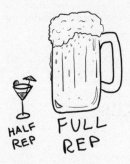

HALF REP   FULL REP

Remember, you lift because you want some stares. You want that attention. But in Tadpole stage, the only time people are going to pay attention to the weight you lift is when you throw on more than you can obviously handle. If you look like you are built from K'nex, people are going to get curious when you start messing around with daddy weight.

They may not necessarily be worried, even though they should be, but they will begin speculating. You can bet dudes are standing on the sidelines asking themselves, "Is this guy really going to lift that? Am I going to have to lift that bar off him? Either way, let me watch in the mirror." Trust me, no one is impressed by how much weight you can re-rack, bro. If you want to earn some respect, then concentrate on a full range of motion and good form. Even though you may not put up real weight for a long time, a little respect is better than no respect. Half-assing more weight than you can handle is far worse than lifting what you can handle properly. Face it, you have a long period ahead of lifting weights that most meatheads use as door stoppers. You have to ride a few ponies before you can run with the bulls. See chapter 10 for a full breakdown of what it means to half rep.

Putting Clips on the Smith Machine

I may not be the smartest guy in the world, but I am the smartest guy in the gym, aka the world. It does not take a whole lot of smarts to know that putting clips on the Smith machine is mythically dumb. This is almost too dumb to believe, but hand to god, I have walked up to a Smith machine

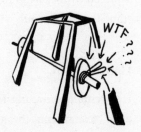

and removed the clips from it. (Now, you are probably wondering why I was even using the Smith machine in the first place, but we all have lapses in judgment. The truth is, I was trying to rip the bar off the Smith machine because all the barbells in the gym were being used.)

Anyway, I appreciate that you are trying to follow gym etiquette. There is nothing more embarrassing than having some loose plates slide off the barbell when you are benching or squatting because your dumb ass forgot to put clips on. But let's just think about this for a second: The only way the weights are going to fall off the Smith machine is if the whole gym flips on its side. Gravity, bro. Use your head.

Curls in the Squat Rack

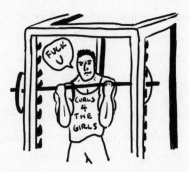

Proceed with caution. The squat rack is a sacred hangout. It is the clubhouse for hard-core Gym Rats, and the moment they see you do your first curl in the squat rack you pretty much become the tender white dude who walks onto the prison yard courts and tries to play soccer with a basketball. Ouch.

There is only one place to do squats: the squat rack. If the squat rack were meant for curls, it would be called "the rest of the gym." If you do not want to ruffle any feathers, the squat rack is not the place to be pumping your guns up for Seth's awesome pool party this weekend.

Shitty Plate Math

Bro, do you even do math? Do you have any sort of instinct for what is right and wrong? Do not ever load up the barbell with plates that add up to the weight of one existing plate. For example, you shouldn't stack on one 25lb plate, a 10lb, and two 5lb plates when you can easily throw on one 45lb plate instead. This looks disgusting. It is paying for a pack of gum with a hundred pennies instead of a dollar; you just look poor. You earned those wagon wheels, so make sure you fucking use them.

The bottom line is, if your weights don't look good, how do you expect to look good?

Using the 2.5lb Plates

Let's say you bench 135lbs and want to get it up to 140lbs. The entire gym is designed around 5lb increments. Introducing a half-pound weight is like introducing the metric system to foot-long sandwiches. When using a barbell, your muscle brain is designed to go up in 10lb increments. There simply is no other way. Introducing a 2.5lb weight is complete anarchy.

BRO MATH: If you keep dividing the weight, you are never going to reach your goal.

Lifting Your Feet Up When You Bench

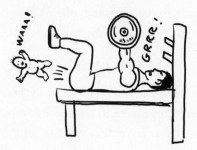

You are grooming yourself to be a CrossFitter by lifting your feet up while you bench. This is extremely disrespectful to the gods who came before you. Bench pressing is a heavy muscle-building exercise, not some froufrou Bosu ball core-tightening Euro cablelaties maneuver. If you are on the bench, aka the king of all exercises, why are you trying to reinvent the wheel? The wheel has already been invented and it comes in cheese form. Or as awesome tiny cars (Hot Wheels).

Leaving Your Blender Ball in Your Shaker

First off, walking around with your shaker cup in the gym says that you have not only been sold on the fact that you need a pre- and post-workout drink, but that you also need to be consuming some sort of supplement on every breath between your sets in order to grow. Now throw in the blender ball and you are screaming, "I will buy any sort of gypsy muscle magic that you feed me!"

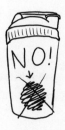

Let's deconstruct this blender ball add-on for a minute. There are three components to a protein shake: protein, water, and a shaker cup. There is one method for creating the shake: Shake the cup. Sure, you may end up with some protein chunks, but if you don't want chunks in your shake then fucking shake it more! Or man up and drink it! If a six-year-old can make chocolate milk without a blender ball, you can make a fucking protein shake without one. What's next? Do you want me to pick the seeds off your strawberries, too, bro?

Chances are that you have done some or all of the above at one point or another in your lifting career, but knowledge is power. Commit this chapter to memory and know that you are only a rookie until you choose not to be. The power is literally in your hands. Follow my steps, and you will go from this to this:

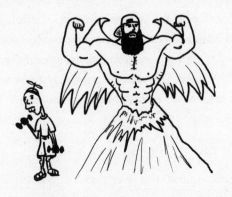

Trust me, there will be a day when you walk into the gym and you'll know you're no longer a rookie. Until then, keep putting up that weight.

CHAPTER 5

Locker Room Etiquette

Believe it or not, there are parts of the gym that have no weights in them. Surprising, I know, but it is equally important to learn how to navigate these foreign waters. The most important one is the locker room. The locker room is where you start and end your gym session, so you better make sure you know your way around.

The locker room is like taking the subway after midnight: Chances are you are going to be fine, but you never know who is going to pull their dick out. If you want to make it out alive, you need to keep all human interaction to a minimum. Trust me, you do not want to accidentally start a conversation with the ass-naked forty-five-year-old divorced dude whose kids hate him. Bro, I see you in the locker room every day, but I never see you in the weight room. Are you just here to creep everybody out? Please do not strike up a conversation with me while you're swinging around your skin slinky. This is not the time to tell me how much you love *Dexter*. The good thing is that after this chapter you will be able to navigate the depths of the locker room at any hour like fucking Magellan. Follow the steps below and Godspeed.

Do Not Be the Naked Guy

What went wrong during your childhood, bro? The locker room is not a fucking nudist colony. Some art student is not sitting three feet away from you trying to paint your gross body. Do you really need to get ass naked before you open your locker or weigh yourself out? I walk into the locker room after crushing a memorable back workout only to see you blow-drying your dick 'fro. Like, everyone is really proud 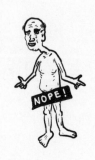 that you are comfortable in your own skin, which looks like raw chicken, but this is not a nude beach, bro. Have some self-respect. And now I know what your bush looks like. Fucking great. How many innocent lives must you ruin?

No Shirt Cocking

In many ways, the shirt cocker is worse than the naked guy. At least the naked guy is committing to something. You, on the other hand, have a body that looks like Grumpy the dwarf's face, and are two steps away from popping up on the sex offender list.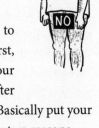

This is the order of operations when it comes to changing into your gym clothes: Take your shirt off first, and put your workout shirt on last. This means put your workout shirt on after your shoes are on and tied, after you take a piss, after you take your pre-workout, etc. Basically put your shirt on as you walk out of the locker room. This is for two reasons:

1. To capitalize on shirtless minutes. Once you start lifting, the times that matter most are those when your shirt is off.

2. Walking around with a shirt on and no pants is sexy when women do it but rapishily creepy for guys. Do not ever shirt cock.

Keep Your Eyes on the Floor

Again, this is exactly like riding on the subway. I know that I am a perfect specimen of a man, but do not stare at me. Staring is what the rest of the gym is for.

Respect the Mirror

The mirror is bodybuilding holy land. The mirror is a shrine to yourself and you pray several times a day, but so does everyone else. Mirror space is limited, so do not waste it with useless activities like shaving, putting your contacts in, or being ugly. After you are done savaging the gym, locker room mirror time is your only chance to be shirtless with a pump in front of a mirror. This is literally the biggest time in your life. Use the opportunity to out-flex your reflection and ask yourself if you compete.

Use a Lock

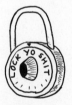

Let's run through the play-by-play: I am juiced up, my skin is itching, and I am ready to commit armed robbery. I am trying to beeline for an open locker and avoid the mob of filthy peasants clawing at my ankles trying to steal my gains, aka regular people. I finally locate what I think is an available locker only to find your dirty shit lying in there.

So I open another locker. Same thing happens, four to five more times. Talk about taking the wind out of my sails. It is personally insulting that you are assuming I will not steal your shit. It is called a *lock*er room. It is not called an "I am an asshole and waste everyone's time because I am too good to lock up my shit" room. By not using a lock, you are tempting fate repeatedly. I have actually met fate. He is fucking huge and will steal your shit. Tread lightly, my friend, tread lightly.

The truth is, when you first start going to the gym, you probably won't use the locker room much anyway. But trust me, as you become more and more of a gym fiend, the locker room will become your second home. You will shower in there, consume various supplements, and store the most important shit you own in your locker. So make sure you take the locker room seriously. It is, after all, part of the Iron Church, and you should show it the respect it deserves.

CHAPTER 6

Should I Take Pre-Workout?

Before we get into this question you should already know the answer to, let me explain exactly what pre-workout is. Pre-workout is a powder developed by scientists to enhance your weightlifting experience. It comes in a variety of flavors and brands, all having one common effect: power.

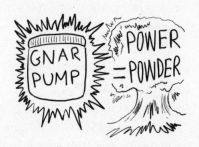

All you have to do is put a scoop of pre-workout in some water, stir it up, and chug it before heading to the gym. This single scoop of pre-workout will hit you with a tingle of energy unlike anything you'll ever experience. So without further ado, let's explore the age-old question of "Should I take pre-workout?"

Let's say you just moved out of your primordial ooze stage and recently started lifting. You put on five pounds of water weight and are already looking for ways to expedite your sick gains, but you do not know where to turn. You are already in the gym hitting arms twice a day, and people can tell you might be a lifter.

Your brofessor can sense that it is time. You have been in the trenches with him and have witnessed him bench more weight than you can calculate. So one day he comes up to you and tells you, "Bro, you have to try this pre-workout. It is fucking nuts. I worked out for four and a half hours and put up three plates on military press then threw up blood in the bathroom for thirty minutes. Superset!" And your response will always be, "Where can I sign up?" You have been drafted. This is World War III and you already won.

Deep down you know that pre-workout is the answer you have been searching for. The first taste of pre-workout is like when Morpheus offers Neo the pill and is like, "Yo, you want to start shooting through walls with your forearm cannons or do you want to be bitch made forever?"

The effects of pre-workout may sound too good to be true, and you would be right to be curious. Let me save you some time. Here are some questions to ask yourself before you take pre-workout:

1. Can I include more powder in my life?
2. Are livers really that important?
3. Do I want to look awesome all the time?
4. Is it safe . . . to look this awesome all the time?
5. Do I have health insurance? Will it cover pre-workout?
6. Do I want to get laid tonight?

If the answer to any of these questions is no, that is fine. Because you're still gonna take pre-workout.

But just to make yourself feel better, you can ask your brofessor some ignorant questions like, "What is in pre-workout?," at which point, your brofessor will glance over the nutritional information and justify any ingredient based on very basic knowledge of other ingredients:

> "Oh, beta alanine? That shit is essential. It's in bread and stuff, so you know it is okay. It makes your muscles do more reps."

> "Creatine monohydrate is found in animals. It is basically in all the meat you eat, so there is no problem with you eating it as powder. My dog eats it, and now so do you."

> "Trimethylglycine is pretty much amino acids. It is all natural and is in plants. Gets you crazy strong, bro."

> "Amino acids? Are you serious, dude? Go back to second grade. Do you know nothing about DNA? Didn't you see *Jurassic* fucking *Park*? Amino acids are why dinosaurs were huge."

As you can see, your brofessor knows what he is talking about. So take the pre-workout, always. Do not concern yourself with consequences. Side effects do not matter to you, which is why they are on the side. The risk of consuming pre-workout is literally outweighed by the weight you lift up after taking it. Now you are ready to take the plunge.

> **BRO TIP:** Do not be a hero. Only start with one scoop of pre. Test your tolerance. I do four scoops, though.

Now, once you take pre-workout, the results can go two different ways. Either your body won't be used to caffeine and you will have too much energy to lift, or you get the sickest, most hyper-focused overly strong lift of your life. Either way it always ends the same: You are going to keep taking pre-workout.

And when months later your brofessor tells you, "Nah, actually the pre-workout was pretty bad for you, because of this ingredient that I am now an expert on. I am on this other pre-workout now," you listen, young brotégé, and you switch up to this new fix.

This is the natural cycle of pre-workouts in your life. They will come and go, but you will always find the next best one to take out for a spin. You never needed a test drive, you just bought the fucking car, crashed it into a telephone pole, ditched it, and got a new one.

So when you ask yourself, "Should I take pre-workout?" just know that the plans were in place long before you arrived. This was a trick question from the start. The pre has you. Just like Morpheus was trying to tell you: You cannot outrun your fate.

CHAPTER 7

You May Now Approach the Bench

The bench is like the president's desk. You cannot just walk in and sit behind it unless you are the leader of the free world. And how do you become president? By putting up some fucking weight.

Let's imagine you walking into the gym for the first time weighing in at 130 pounds, soaking wet. You just wandered into the wrong hood, my friend. This is scary shit. This is *Training Day* and I am Denzel and you are that white dude who smoked PCP. The question is, how are you going to handle the situation once you step into this unfamiliar territory? Well, you are going to communicate the only way you know how: You are going to hit the bench. The bench is the universal language. The bench is caveman shit.

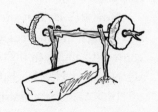

You think Tom Hanks would have needed to build a raft to get off that island if he just had a better bench? No. He would have swum his way home.

If you are here to get big, which you are, you need to treat the gym like the church that it is. If you are here to tone up for the summer or check in on Facebook, I suggest you start on the elliptical—you know, that plastic thing with the skis that puts cotton in your biceps. But for someone serious about getting huge, the answer is go big or go home. In my case, I do not have a home because my mom kicked me out of hers for growing weed in the basement, so I only have one option, and that is to bench.

Now, when it comes to finding a vacant bench, let's be real with each other for a second. The chances of you walking into the gym and finding an empty bench are slimmer than that chick you dry fingered on the dance floor actually texting you back. If you expect to walk into the gym to find a nice, quiet, open bench, then you are in Candy Land, my friend. You are looking for the Easter Bunny. It is a myth. It does not exist.

The bench is, and always will be, the hottest item in the gym. The bench is Tickle Me Elmo in '96. So you can bet you will have to wrestle a few soccer moms to the ground before getting your hands on one.

Listen, on any given day, everyone in the gym is hitting chest. You can walk into 24 Hour Fitness at 3:00 A.M. on Saturday, drunk, thinking, "Oh, nobody is here so I am going to smack my chest around," and you would be wrong, because everybody is here and they are all hitting chest.

Now, let's say that after days of walking past the crowded benches and doing weird stalker loops around the gym, you finally build up the courage to approach the bench, where it turns out Vin Diesel is mid-set. No sweat. Here is what you do: Wait for him to rack the bar and sit up. This means he is finished with his set and ready for compliments. Now is your in. Approach the bench with your sack tucked back and say these exact words in the softest voice you can: "Excuse me, how many sets do you have left?" This is a pointless question. He could have thirty sets left and you are still going to wait for the bench, but the key is that you established that you are next. This is no different than walking into a local pool hall and slapping some quarters on the edge of the table.

Now be prepared for at least fifteen minutes of awkward standing around, pretending you are stretching while you wait. Be patient—your time will come. This is a good time to get some Tinder swipes in.

Okay, it is go time. Now you are at the plate. Take a second to look around. There are mirrors everywhere. The bench is center stage. It is finally time to dress up the bar. She is naked, so throw some clothes on her and make her look nice. You are like Richard Gere in *Pretty Woman* and you are going to fuck the shit out of this bar.

When it comes to bench pressing, anything less than a 45lb plate on each side of the barbell is an insult to the bench and to Bro Science itself. But if this is your first time benching, you are not going to throw up wagon wheels like it's the Oregon Trail. People will judge you.

BRO TIP: If you cannot bench at least 135lbs, lift with a bro who can put up at least 225lbs. This will make up for the lack of weight you can put up. Now no one will fuck with you because they know you are being learned. You are protected by Bro Science.

Now it is time to silence the haters.

Lie down, put your feet on the floor, grab the bar, and bang it out! This is like the first time you hit it doggy style. Do not worry about going for time—go for pure speed. Chances are you only have four to five reps in you anyway.

How did that feel? You do not need to answer that, because it felt fucking awesome. You just established yourself in the gym pecking order. Now others can see you, and all you want to do is make them see more of you. You still have a long way to go before you are president, but the path to the Swolval Office has been laid out in front of you.

CHAPTER 8

How to Deadlift

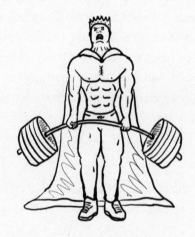

The deadlift is the king of all lifts, which means it must be treated with respect. It is an advanced lift where form is most important.

There is possibility for injury when it comes to this movement, so do not prance up to the bar and try to yank 135lbs just because you watched a couple of YouTube instructional videos about it. Believe me, I get it, I know how shredded I look when you see me deadlift. It's insane. Every fiber of muscle is about to burst through the skin, they are getting worked so hard. You will get there.

Since deadlifts are the lift of kings, allow me to begin with a quote from Ronnie Coleman, aka black Jesus, aka regular Jesus: "Everybody want to be a bodybuilder, but don't nobody wants to lift no heavy-ass weight." The same goes for deadlifts. Everybody wants to deadlift but don't nobody want to deadlift. The last thing you want is to fuck up, look like a noob, and throw your back out. I see you walking into the gym thinking you are hot shit, only to approach the deadlift platform looking like a fucking peasant. Don't front.

The first step in learning how to deadlift is to whip your dick out and ask the world if it wants to suck it. In other words, ask your lifting buddy if he wants to deadlift today, hoping he will say no, but he says yes and now you have to deadlift. Face it: At some point everybody has got to die.

> **BRO TIP:** Always deadlift with a bro. Deadlifting alone is like trying to get pussy sober. You do not have the confidence for this. You are not going to pull any tail and you are not going to pull any weight. The only thing you are going to pull is the rip cord and head to the dumbbell rack to lift arms.

Deadlifting is an ideal gym buddy lift, especially when you are starting out. You want your gym buddy to harshly critique your form so you get it down perfectly. There is no room for error here. There is also a lot of assembly and disassembly to the deadlift. You are going to be walking back and forth with 45lb plates, slapping them onto the barbell, and removing them repeatedly. This process takes time. Cut that time in half with a gym buddy, and get this show on the road.

Now, theoretically, you can deadlift anywhere there is space for a barbell. And theoretically you can fuck anything that has space for your dick, but that is not an open invite for you to come over and jack off into my bath towels. Deadlifting in the free weight area? What are you, a fucking savage? There are only two acceptable places to deadlift:

Outside of the Squat Rack

Do not deadlift inside the squat rack. Since you are deadlifting, the loaded-up barbell should be resting on the floor, therefore making it unnecessary for you to be inside of the squat rack. You will get blacklisted for misusing squat rack space. So instead of taking up space there, move the bar outside the rack.

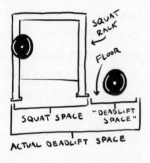

Now, technically, you are not taking up the squat rack even though you are technically taking up even more space. And that's perfectly fine because you are fucking deadlifting. No one is going to mess with you.

The Deadlift Platform

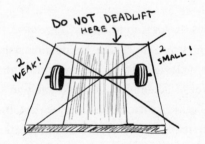

This is an area specifically designed for deadlifts, but do not be fooled. You cannot deadlift here. The deadlift platform is high-stakes poker. Do not sit at the table with your broke ass unless you have chips to move. Unless the gym is completely empty and you have a guarantee that no one will be entering for the rest of the day, or you can deadlift at least 315lbs, you cannot use the deadlift platform.

Okay, now that you have your deadlift all set up, do a thorough warm-up of zero to four reps of just the bar. Do not warm up with any weight on the bar, because once you put weight on the bar people will assume that you are now lifting. After your warm-up of nothing, throw on your maximum and minimum weight, which is the same, because again, you are a noob.

Next is grip. There are four ways to grip the bar for deadlifts—three of which you should do, two of which you can do, and one of which you will do.

In the first grip, we are going to eliminate straps.

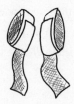

Straps are useful when you have reached the point when you can deadlift literally more weight than you can hold, and that is a long way off. Sure, you can lift heavier if you use straps, but you know what else makes you lift heavier? Getting stronger. Which you are not going to do if you use straps right off the bat. Using straps when you start dead-lifting is like using a Fleshlight the first time you jerk off. Yeah, it makes it better, but who are you, Inspector Gadget? Use your goddamn hands like a fucking man.

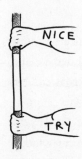

Next to go is overhand regular grip.

Overhand regular grip is a fairy tale. Your grip strength is worse than the claw game at the carnival. Any prize worth pulling is going to slip right out.

Third is hook grip.

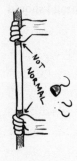

You found out about hook grip way too late and now it just feels wrong. Hook grip is like trying to learn a second language. What is the point of learning a second language if you already have a first one?

And by process of elimination, we have over-under grip.

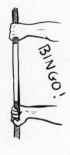

Over-under grip is your only dance move; your home run swing. The only minor issue with over-under grip is potential long-term muscle imbalance. You will think to yourself, "Do I have to switch my grip every set to even out my muscles? What if I am doing three sets? Do I have to do four sets now? I didn't even want to deadlift today. Where the dumbbells at?" Welcome to the club.

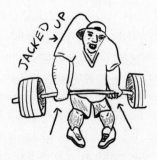

Moving on. I am going to skip form altogether since you most likely will as well. There are entire encyclopedia volumes dedicated to deadlift form, but I'm not a fucking librarian. Check that shit out yourself.

Next up is banging the weights. In a proper deadlift, the weights should be banging against the floor. Does this mean you should be slamming 135lbs like you're building a fucking railroad? No, fuck off, John Henry. Making noise in the gym is a privilege, not a right. If you are not pulling a bare minimum of 315lbs, then the only thing I should be able to hear is the sound of you queefing mid-set.

At the end of the day, if you are like me and you fucking hate following instructions, then just shut up and deadlift. After all, it's better to die on your feet than lift on your knees.

CHAPTER 9

Dumbbell (Dombell) Curls

Listen, there are going to be days when you just do not feel like lifting. Maybe you got all hyped up to wreck chest then walked into the gym at 5:30 P.M. on a Wednesday and saw a line long enough to kill Rick James twice. Maybe your boy got a full-time offer from that sick sales job he hates, and you had ten too many tequila shots the night before to celebrate. Or maybe you just want to lift the only body parts that instantly get pumped to remind yourself of what greatness looks like.

In an ideal world, your weekly gym split would look like this:

Monday: chest

Tuesday: back

Wednesday: legs

Thursday: shoulders

Friday: arms

Saturday and Sunday: hard-core day drinking

-◖—◖-

Once you actually start lifting, your split is going to look more like mine:

Monday: chest and triceps

Tuesday: back and biceps

Wednesday: shoulders

Thursday: arms

Friday: chest and arms

Saturday: back and arms

Sunday: attempt legs, do biceps

The reality of the situation is that your arms are the holder of the glory pump, and once you see that rock swole happening in front of your own eyes, you will get hooked. It is live-action television and you are the fucking star. The biceps are the boners of the arms, after all. Eventually, you will get to the point where you cannot leave the gym without sneaking in a few sets of dumbbell curls. You will develop an addiction that will only get worse, and that is just fine. Every single day is arm day.

Here's why that happens, according to a very prominent Bro Science theory. When you walk into the gym, you are cold and you are dry. There are mirrors everywhere, and you feel fucking small. The next thing you know, you catch your reflection and immediately become paranoid that you shrunk, so you beeline it for the dumbbell rack, sneak in a few curls, and snag yourself a pump. Oh, looks like you got your swagger back. You are back on the radar. What it boils down to is that without a pump, you are a nobody. It is that simple. There is no other part of your body capable of catching a pump as quickly as your biceps.

In addition to being the quickest way to feel swole, the great thing about dumbbell curls is how transportable they are. Let's say that you are on the way to the leg press. No problem, carpool some dumbbells and superset legs with dumbbell curls. Put the blood back where it belongs and restore order in your body. Have you ever wondered why the 35lb dumbbells are always missing? It's because people are hoarding them so they can do bicep curls between their sets. There is something about curling 35lbs that just seems right. 35lbs dumbbells are just heavy enough, but they are not so heavy that you are going to have to actually try.

If you really think about it, bicep curls are not an exercise, they are a tool. You aren't wrecking your biceps for overall strength, movement, or to break a sweat. You are lifting biceps to get that rock swole.

Let's go over the bicep curl movement. The first step is to grab some dumbbells off the rack. When you are grabbing them, do not look at what you are doing, just stare at your forearms. Now stand in front of the mirror with your arms at your sides, chest up, shoulders back, and *turn on the forklift.*

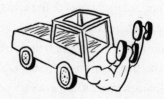

Stare at your biceps in the mirror until they stare back.

BRO TIP: Curl with your palm up to get that softball in your arm. Make sure to stare at the dude next to you. Make sure he sees your pump. You are alpha.

Unlike the bench press, when it comes to bicep curls, there is no pride in your weight. Curls are not about the weight, they are about the pump. You could be swinging around 65lb dumbbells, but everyone will be thinking, "Who are you trying to impress, bro?" If you are repping out on 15lb dumbbells with a sick pump, I won't even have anything bad to say to you. Remember the golden rule of Bro Science:

It is not about how much you can lift, but about how much it looks like you can lift.

Now, when it comes to standing vs. sitting during bicep curls . . . this is a hot debate. I recommend you stand up when you curl to maximize that mirror space, but I never follow my own advice, which is why I sit and curl, and why I have three DUIs. Any chance I have to take a seat and work out, I take. Give me a break, I am working out over here.

It's time to put on a show. Grab two tickets to the blood circus and have your boy film the show and post that shit to Instagram immediately! #ArmedRobbery.

CHAPTER 10

Don't Be a Half Repper

Earlier in *The Swoly Bible* I mentioned how much of a rookie mistake half repping is, but the truth is this major gym offense deserves its own chapter. If you are caught half repping in the gym, chances are no one will say anything, but that's because everyone has given up on you. Luckily, I am here to be your Swoly Spirit and remind you of the rights and wrongs of the Iron Church.

No matter your level of participation, lifting is a lifestyle based around showing off. If it is your first day touching iron, I guarantee you will try to look tougher than you ever have before. If you are a professional competition lifter, you are lifting to literally compete in a show-off contest. If you are just a regular-ass bro (you are) then you are lifting to show off at beaches and bars in front of other regular-ass bros. In the weight room, your ego and your body are literally inflated while you lift heavy weight and stare at yourself in a mirror, which is why you love lifting. And because everyone in the gym is a professional show-off, you are not fooling anyone when you throw on more weight than you can handle and barely complete a full rep. Half repping is an easy trap to fall into, so it is vital that you define your habit before it defines you.

Half repping is when a guy bullshits his way through 225lbs on bench, and acts like he is now part of the 225lb club. That is personally insulting. If you have ever made it to the point where you can properly rep out 225lbs on bench, you know that feeling of accomplishment. You have been down that long and dark and hideous road of 185lbs and 205lbs, benching those weights for what felt like an eternity. Now this asshole hops on the bench, carelessly throws on two plates, struggles to unrack it, bends his elbows a few times, then sits up and acts like he is your fucking bro. Fuck that. Half reppers have no respect for the weight because they have no respect for themselves.

And yo, listen, this is serious. You may be a half repper and not even know it. You may find yourself spouting heresy like, "You should only go down until your elbows are at 90 degrees on bench or else it is bad for your shoulders." You are basically the equivalent of the guy that claims your dick only needs to be three inches because that is all a vagina can feel. Bullshit and you know it. (It is two and a half inches, anyway.) So if you suspect you or a friend might be a half repper, be a good muscle friend and call the police, aka the swolice, immediately. Here are four of America's Most Wanted:

Bad Benching Billy

WANTED FOR: Not touching the bar to his chest on bench press. Bench loitering.

LAST SEEN: Stacking on plates with no clips, stalling for attention, then proceeding to struggle to bend his elbows approximately 30 degrees before slamming weight back onto rack. The suspect was then reported to sit up and claim, "Nailed it," and continued to recklessly add more weight.

KNOWN ASSOCIATES: Squad of bench bros inciting a douche riot of high fives and poor form. And an overly involved spotter.

Half Squatting Harry

WANTED FOR: Not squatting to at least parallel, thinking he is better than you just because he is "lifting" legs.

LAST SEEN: In the squat rack repeatedly swinging under the bar. Flagrant grunts were heard and a disturbance was reported as community members complained that "there is no way he is actually going to squat that." Eyewitness testimony claims a squat descension of no more than five inches. Onlookers were horrified as the suspect's shaky knees re-racked the bar. Half Squatting Harry was last seen wearing knee wraps, a lifting belt, and a beer gut.

KNOWN ASSOCIATES: Band of middle-aged married men who just want to get out of the house for an hour. And a dangerously unqualified spotter who is unmarried and possibly a little gay.

Pussy Pull-Up Pete

WANTED FOR: Violent use of momentum during pull-ups, rep counterfeiting, and thinking those were actually pull-ups.

LAST SEEN: Holding the cable machine hostage. Eyewitness reports of erratic behavior in the form of a bullshit push-up, burpee, pull-up circuit. Heavy casualties sustained due to European levels of excessive sweat spray.

KNOWN ASSOCIATES: A misfit gang of unfit CrossFitters and the "sports rehabilitation" dude who is constantly peddling his unlicensed massage therapy sessions.

Cheat Curl Chad

WANTED FOR: Falsifying strength reports, illegal use of the squat rack, and trespassing on mirror real estate.

LAST SEEN: In a heated altercation with uninterested gymgoers. Eyewitnesses speculated a dispute arose from Chad's inability to curl

135lbs. Suspect considered not known to be armed and is definitely not dangerous. Charges of being a major douchebag pending.

KNOWN ASSOCIATES: None.

—⬤———⬤—

If you have witnessed any of the above muscle crimes or have any information on the whereabouts of these suspects, it is your civic duty to enforce the code of Bro Science. Please Tweet any photographic evidence to @Brosciencelife #HalfRepper.

CHAPTER 11

Yo, Can I Get a Spot?

Learning how to properly spot another lifter is a lesson often overlooked in the lifting community. Being taught how to spot is like being taught how to pay your taxes once you get out of college: It is not taught, it is learned through harsh real-world realities.

Google defines spotting as "the act of supporting another person during a particular exercise, with an emphasis on allowing the participant to lift or push more than they could normally do safely." Dom defines spotting as: getting a few more muscle reps out of your bro that he didn't know he had.

Spotting is the closest thing to a relationship that you've ever had.

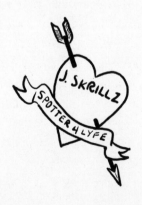

Spotting is communication; spotting is trust; it is understanding yourself and your spotter physically and mentally. Spotting is grunting, and sweating, and heavy breathing, and accomplishment, all condensed into fifteen seconds.

The moment you set foot in the gym, you are expected to know how to spot your gym buddy. And when that moment arrives, you have to jump right into the role, because you are not about to bail on your bro. Spotting is the only safety measure in the gym, but there is nothing safe about trying to max out at 405lbs for the first time ever with a 130-pound dude spotting you. You better believe the guy you are spotting is thinking, "Bro, can you make sure this 350lb barbell does not crush my neck and cut my head clean off?" while you hover over him.

Now, if you are sitting all alone on the bench and feel like putting up some weight that you know you cannot put up and you don't have your gym buddy with you, let's talk about how to find that spot. That lifeline.

The first step is to load up your weight to the point where it is obvious that you need a spotter; to the point of danger. Next, sit on the end of your bench, survey the scene and look for a civilian (ideally without headphones) who is trying to kill time. You need to try to look like you are not just a piece of shit hogging the bench and swinging your arms around. Now once you locate your dude, your mate, the one that meets all of your qualifications, it is time to force eye contact with him and make your presence felt. Forcing eye contact is already in your wheelhouse from all of your creepy attempts at seducing chicks at the bar. So once your spotter sees you, make it seem like he was the one that noticed you first. This process is the awkward mating dance, the "So can I buy you a drink?" of the gym.

Now, here is the tip to the guy being spotted: Do not try to impress your spotter. You just dragged this innocent bystander from the middle of his sick back workout to spot your bony ass. Just because you now have a spotter does not mean that you can slap on all the 45lb plates in the gym. Your spotter is hovering over you, praying you do not say, "Hey, now that you are here, I am going to go for, like, 450lbs or 500lbs." Fuck you. This guy just watched you struggle with 185lbs. Do not make the poor dude load up a bunch of plates just to see you fail. Your spotter knows he is going be doing all of the work from rep one and you are going to sit up and act like you almost had it. No spotter wants to end up deadlifting the bar off your chest. Well, actually if he is ripping back, then he might. Either way, do not abuse the privilege of having a spotter.

Here Are Some Dos and Don'ts for the Spotter

- Do not be a bitch. Do be a muscle friend. Do not act like this is a major inconvenience for you even though it definitely is. No lifter hitting bench wants to look up and see some pissed-off spotter staring down at him literally holding his life in his hands.

- When you grab a bar, grab it evenly with an over-under grip. Do not randomly pick a spot on one side of the bar and yank on it, or else you are going to be half-helping and half-crushing the guy who's lifting. When he started his set, the bar was perfectly balanced. Keep it that way. I do not know anything about physics, but I do know that if you don't grab the bar evenly, you are an asshole.

- Do stand close enough to the bench with one foot forward so you are able to lift some heavy weight if needed. Do not stand directly over the dude you are spotting dangling your balls over his forehead. He is about to put up some serious poundage and does not want to be mouth breathing your sack scent through it.

- Do not be the spotter who panics at the first sight of struggle and tears the weight from the dude's hands when he had at least three more reps in him. Any spaz like this is a gain thief of a spotter. You are never going to get those reps back. You just spent your rent money on gym membership and supplements, and now this dude is stealing your gains? What did you do to deserve this?

- Do not be the spotter who thinks he is going to get one more rep by leaving the bar on your chest and screaming at you. Screaming, "You got one more!" does not mean that I am going to manufacture the ATP in my muscles and get this bar to move. If the bar is on its way back down, that is the opposite of one more. This is also the opposite of helping. Fail.

- Last and most important, after a successful spot, let the lifter sit up and ask you how much you helped. Regardless of the truth, you must tell him that the lift was "All him." Then celebrate and talk about how much weight he is going to put up next time.

Congratulations, you have conducted your first successful spot. You have contributed back to society in the most meaningful way possible: by making it stronger. You have committed a selfless act; you should feel good about yourself. Actually, maybe you shouldn't . . . your left trap looks a little deflated, bro.

CHAPTER 12

Whey Too Much Brotein

> **BRO FACT:** Proteins are like Legos. Protein is the building block of muscle; Legos are the building blocks of building blocks. Ipso facto, you can never have enough of either.

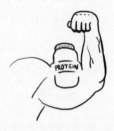

When it comes to protein, there are a ton of options out there, so you gotta make sure you pick the right one. Protein is your best friend. Protein is your brotein. Lucky for you, I am here to narrow your proteins down to the best type to fit your lifting style.

There are a ton of brands of whey protein out there. It can definitely be complicated to narrow it down, so let me make it easy for you. Always go with Optimum. Optimum is a quality protein, but quality does not matter. What does matter is that my bro told me that Optimum was the best when I first started lifting. I never asked him why, and I never stopped believing him. Optimum has been in the game since the jump. It is grassroots shit. Optimum is honest. Optimum is part of the culture. Optimum says, "Hey, I fucking lift. I'm not here to waste my time doing bullshit workouts and looking pretty." That's a look you want.

A good rule to remember when it comes to choosing a protein is if it seems too good to be true, then it probably is. If your protein tastes like milkshakes, then it's time to reconsider. Check the ingredients on the canister to make sure it isn't less than 50 percent pure. If the contents are 50 percent protein and 50 percent incinerated Snickers bars, it's not worth the money. You should be leasing a Civic, bro; not buying an M6. If you do get an M6, hit me up, though.

Don't be afraid to judge proteins by their covers. Read the names of them. Does the name just sound expensive? That's because it probably is. If the price tag is more expensive than Kim Kardashian's tit milk, then you don't need to cram this necessary expense into your muscle budget. Trust me, you will always find that one dude who will preach that expensive protein brand to you and you will immediately stop listening to him. This is the same guy who goes to Equinox and crushes the Smith machine. Yeah, all right, buddy. See you in church.

Flavor

Now let us move on to the flavor of protein. The question is: Can you judge someone based on the flavor of protein they consume? The answer is: Absolutely.

Let's say you buy strawberry banana flavor. You immediately have others thinking, "Bro, do you even lift?" Strawberry banana flavored protein exists to filter out people who do not lift. If you are prancing around drinking pink liquid, then you are probably the dude doing machine circuits. Chocolate or die, bro.

If sometimes you get a little tired of chocolate and want to mix it up, you can get away with snagging some vanilla and mixing in some

OJ, but mixing protein is not *Breaking Bad*, it is Bro Science, so just stick to chocolate.

Value

When it comes to calculating the value of your protein I have a master's in Economics, Chemistry, and Bation. Masturbation.

There are no two ways around it: Protein is expensive. Drinking protein is like drinking money. There are three points to be considered in finalizing your choice of protein: price, servings, and grams per serving. Check the stats on the label and make sure that you are receiving enough protein with enough servings for the coin you are about to drop. Fuck retirement accounts, put your cash into what really grows.

Once you find the protein that is right for you, make sure to drink your body weight in it every day. People might try to tell you that you shouldn't drink too much protein, cuz it might make you fat or fuck up your stomach, yada yada yada. These are the exact same people who are going to tell you not to bench every day as a warm-up. Do not listen to these haters. Get your weight up by getting your scoops up. Give it a month, and watch as they come crawling back and ask you how you got so fucking yoked. Obtaining the mass you want isn't only about pushing past your plateaus in the gym, it's also about consuming a shitload of protein and then some more for dessert.

STAGE 3

Brotégé

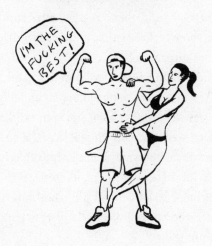

The Brotégé stage begins approximately six months after you start lifting. At this point, you have maxed out your beginner gains and finally have a hint of muscle. These minuscule gains go straight to your head, which is what is supposed to happen. You have officially crossed over to the other side.

Now, it may not be clear to you, but to everyone else, you are by no means big. But they can hate all they want; their opinion does not mean shit to you, because you are now a brotégé. The Brotégé stage is the first and only time that you will actually think you are big, because body dysmorphia has not set in yet. I am so jealous. Body dysmorphia is the number-one cause of getting huge and the number-one cause of feeling forever small. It's an endless cycle. It's like opening up new credit cards to pay the debt on your old ones.

Of all the stages of your lifting evolution, your confidence will be at its peak during the Brotégé stage. You look in the mirror and actually see mass, chicks start to take notice of you, and you've even found yourself voluntarily offering gym noobs unwanted advice. You are like that star varsity quarterback's younger brother who never got any attention and ran track, and then emerges after summer break with some facial hair, some fucking gains, and swagger dripping off his Air Maxes. Do not act surprised, bro.

Now you understand why you got into this game. Welcome to the court, LeBron. You just won rookie of the year and it is only game one. Whoa, you just signed onto Facebook and your ex liked your new prof pic? Ego win. Last weekend you tongue kissed a couple of chicks at your hometown bar during your summer break? Wrong. You tongue kissed three and did some over-the-pants stuff. You are the shit.

Enjoy the Brotégé stage while it lasts, hotshot. It is all about the confidence effect. Study the following chapters to truly take advantage of your fifteen minutes.

CHAPTER 13

How to Find a Gym Buddy

Congratulations, you are now going to the gym every day by yourself without looking like a complete rookie. You have a basic understanding of gym etiquette and know your way around almost every piece of gym equipment. Last week you put up 135lbs on the bench for two reps with no spotter, which was awesome, but you knew you had a couple more reps in you. We've all been here. You feel alone, but you have a suspicion that there's someone out there that you haven't met yet, but who could very well be right in front of you.

If you have been a lifting cowboy since college, then your biological clock is probably ticking and you are thinking it is time to settle down. Here are some Bro Tips on how to find the one. The one more rep you did not know you had in you . . . until your gym buddy told you that you did.

Working In

Working in is a common gym occurrence that happens when an individual is using a piece of equipment and another person asks to use the machine between his/her sets. The correct way to phrase this question is simple: "Mind if I work in?" If executed properly, working in is a great way to make a gym buddy, but it's all about making sure you work in the right way, so you don't end up creeping out a potential muscle swoldier. This isn't Tinder, bro. Stop coming on so strong.

When you head to the gym, you have laser focus and want the rest of the gym to know that. You lift with intention, headphones blaring the newest Tiësto song and a look on your face that tells the world not to fuck with you. But deep down, we both know you want a gym buddy, and working in is an easy way to let your guard down. Imagine it is back day and you are deadlifting in the squat rack because you are too lazy to finagle the bar from out of the cage. Say it is your first set, and you have already stacked on 315lbs (because warm-ups are for pussies), when some bro comes over looking like he could be your Venom. He asks how many sets you got left. You have three, but you tell him you got two, because you are immediately on the defensive. You politely offer him the option to work in with you, because that is the right thing to do. You assume he wants to squat and he will decline your offer because he will not want to rearrange the weight you already have on the bar.

Joke is on you, hotshot. It turns out this guy is deadlifting, too, and he accepts your bullshit offer. To demonstrate your alpha-ness, you ask if he wants to take some of the weight off. He says, "Nah, it's fine."

BRO FACT: You just became best friends. He successfully deadlifts your weight and you two end up doing the entire workout together.

This is awesome. This random dude lifts the same as you, he looks the same as you, but your chest is definitely a little bigger and you are probably stronger than him on certain lifts, too. You exchange numbers and make a promise to hit chest and triceps tomorrow. This is the closest you will get to workout serendipity.

Fresh Meat

Recruit a civilian who does not lift to start lifting, just so you have a spot. The CrossFit section of the gym is a great place to look, but be cautious, as there are risks to this. It is like hooking up with a chick who is still a virgin. Sure, you get to show off your experience, but she might have a fuckload of dependency issues. On the plus side, your new gym buddy is going to do whatever you want to do. But once you have been lifting together for a while, he will not know how to lift (live) without you. He will follow you around relentlessly, constantly asking you questions and hitting you up to get a lift in. Maybe you are out to dinner with your bros and all of a sudden a glass of champagne gets delivered to you by "the gentleman sitting alone at the bar." Just saying, it could happen. Finally, you tell him to chill the fuck out because you need your space. Then you cut the cord and notice he bleached his hair and is doing exercises with poor form, trying to get your attention. Eventually he stops lifting and gets fat . . . whatever, as long as he is happy (he's not).

The Complimenter

The complimenter is the dude who will sneak up on you during your set, pinch your shoulder, and tell you how sick your gains are, and then insist you work out together. You nod your head over and over and hope that he goes away. This dude has no concept of social structure. He is like that creepy dude at the club who comes out of nowhere and tells a chick she is the most beautiful girl in the world and demands they get married.

The Student

Find a guy who needs your advice. You might think a lot of dudes don't need your advice, but they all do, because Bro Science has no end, because you can never be big enough. Start by lifting close to him and making your presence felt, but not doing anything so sudden as to startle him. Wait for him to finish his set and offer a gentle yet completely unsolicited piece of advice like, "Yo, you ever try tilting your hands down when you do lateral raises? Like you are showering some sorority chicks in champagne." And then impress and confuse him with hard-to-pronounce scientific terms like, "Make sure to squeeze your shoulder blades together; keep your scapula rotini nice and al dente." He will have no idea that you are full of shit and neither will you. But he will be intrigued and you might just find yourself a new gym buddy.

Study Buddy

Find an empty bench, load up your weight, and scan the gym for a dude you think could be a good gym friend. Then ask him for a spot for the sole purpose of starting a conversation.

Spotting is necessary and the most casual way of forcing interaction. It is like asking a chick to come over and study—you might need the help, but getting an A is not why you invited her over. Same goes with this. You could use this spot, but you probably were not maxing out anyway. Once you have the dude spotting you, don't miss your opportunity. When your set is done and he tells you, "It was all you, bro," don't hesitate to ask him what he does for chest. Just like that chick you invited over to study, lifters can't turn down unwarranted compliments.

Lurking Louie

On the other hand, you can also make yourself extra available for spots. Look for a dude getting ready for a heavy lift. Read the signs. He will be scanning the gym and stalling. This is an opportunity; someone has to spot him, so make sure it is you. You are that guy who pounces on a chick as soon as she becomes single on Facebook. Catch 'em at a moment of weakness. The guy's probably got this, but maybe he is questioning his confidence. Who is going to be there for him? You are. Sure, the Lurking Louie method is a little creepy and kind of pathetic, but it is effective nonetheless. You think a hyena gives a shit if it's preying off a wounded animal? Hell, no.

Listen, your lifting career is just like a relationship. There are going to be ups and downs—times when your gym buddy will want to see other people, involve others in your setup, or bail on you completely. Don't matter to you, though, because you now know all the ways to find a new buddy and make your old one jealous. Boom.

CHAPTER 14

How to Take a Selfie

Man, it is just one of those days. One of those good days that Ice Cube had, except yours is better and you used your AKs, your arm kannons.

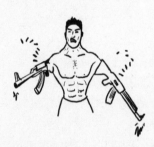

You have been having more and more of these days. You woke up looking shredded as fuck because you're dehydrated from getting hammered last night. You don't even have a hangover because you got home, did a drunk full body circuit in your bedroom at 4:30 A.M., and threw up in your roommate's closet. You feel strong. You rip a few egg whites, chug some Gnar Pump, and hustle over to the gym to crush one of the best lifts to date.

After you have completed a swole session, what is the first thing you do? Drink a protein shake? Wrong. You unholster your iPhone and take a fucking selfie. Listen, if you do not post at least one selfie within thirty minutes of achieving a nasty pump, you will immediately and unmercifully lose all your gains. This is known as the anabolic window.

Here are some tips on how to take the perfect swelfie and harvest mad likes because Instagram likes are anabolic. When it comes to getting likes on Instagram, you can call me Lichael Jordan. Once you become big enough, Instagram and Facebook are no longer social media, they are *mass* media.

Where to Take the Selfie

The optimal location to take your selfie is the locker room. Just think about it; we are talking about easy access to full-length mirrors when your pump is so fresh that it still has the sticker on it. However, there are two problems with the locker room.

Some people, aka haters, might not be happy about you snapping pictures of yourself while their dicks are out. Pay these people no mind. Do you.

When you are new to swelfies, you may be insecure about snapping one with an audience. But you gotta start somewhere, so you try to sneak a quick one.

Lighting

Fitness is 98 percent lighting; the other 2 percent is the sun effect on Instagram. You may be wondering how to tell if you have located the best lighting or not, and that is the right question to be asking. Finding good lighting is all trial and error. It takes endless practice, but once you have mastered the process you will have an appreciation for light unlike anyone else. While your friends are doing weird shit like having a conversation during brunch, you will be snapping fifteen to one hundred of the best-lit selfies imaginable. One of these selfies is definitely going to at least break dub-digit likes on the 'gram. Also, why the fuck are you at brunch? Inhale some tuna straight out of the can and get to the gym.

When it comes to lighting, not even Bud or Miller can pinpoint the factors involved that make you look shredded, and those dudes invented light. There is not a single thing you can do to create good lighting because you have to find it. But rest assured that you will not ever find light; light will find you, and when the light finds you, you will know it, and when you know it, you take a selfie.

How to Take the Selfie

At this point, you have at least twenty-five variations of the same pose and facial expression down. Run through each of them and decide which pose is your moneymaker for the day. Now, it does not matter which body part you worked out that day because you are going to flex all of your muscles, even the ones you cannot flex, like your teeth and your brain. This massive body flex will come together to form the aesthetic symphony that you are going to post straight to Instagram and push to Facebook, duh. Make sure not to forget your order of operations: PEMDAS: Peep Every Muscle Dat Are Swole.

Before we get into the step-by-step process of creating that perfect swelfie, prepare yourself. You are going to sink thirty minutes into capturing the perfect picture, experiencing extreme fatigue and heavy breathing from flexing all your muscles while holding your breath; you are going to get mad blurry pictures caused by hands shaky from trying to hold a phone camera steady while flexing and not breathing; and you will get cramps, because you are supersetting your workout with a total body workout, and not breathing. That is all. You will get used to it.

STEP ONE

Inhale, flex your abs, and hold your breath. You are going to be holding your breath for a long time. You will become so good at holding your breath you should get an honorary diver's certificate.

STEP TWO

Flex your lat into your non-phone hand. This will make you appear wider and your arm appear bigger.

STEP THREE

Commence open-hand flex of the arm. The absence of a fist will achieve that natural, "I swear I'm not flexing" look. Even though everyone knows that you are flexing and posing, you want to do your best to make the pose look natural. Eventually this will become your normal physical state, which is something to look forward to.

STEP FOUR

Bring the phone up in a slow, hammer curl motion. Initiate arm flex. Do not rush this. Make sure to get that grapefruit in your bicep, bro.

STEP FIVE

Engage chest muscles, maintain all other muscles in flexed position. At this point you may start shaking, but push through. It will be worth it.

STEP SIX

Activate hard-face. Look concerned. Think RoboCop. Stare at your phone, never at the mirror. Ace the hard-face and your Instagram is going to be flooded with DMs from bodybuilding blogs asking you to model for their account. Your dreams are getting closer and your muscles are getting bigger. Planets are approaching alignment.

STEP SEVEN

Frame up the shot, steady the phone, and prepare for art. You are about to take countless swelfies, each more valuable than the one before. Years from now, these pieces will be auctioned for millions. You have made an everlasting contribution to humanity; give yourself a pat on the back.

After you have sifted through your seventy-five pictures and arrived at today's featured photo, it is time to make magic happen. Post that shit to Instagram and get those likes that keep your ass in the gym. Always make sure that your hashtags are solid. Your fans need to know that you are #dedicated, #shreddedcheddar, #cleanandlean, #gymtitan, etc., because without hashtags, how are people supposed to know what you stand for? Certainly not by the picture you just posted. Listen, a picture is worth a thousand hashtags, so make sure to put a thousand hashtags.

Now that you're blasting through the Brotégé stage, you are starting to realize that you are more than just a gym bro. You are a spectacle. You are the poster child for hard work, dedication, and change. You are doing your country a disservice by not sharing your progress with the rest of us. So if you ever have any thoughts running through your head like, "Man, I just spent an hour trying to take this swelfie and I still can't get the right light, maybe I should give up," DON'T. Go back to the gym, bang out some curls, and let the light find you. And if that still doesn't work, throw a fuckin' filter on that bad boy and hit share.

CHAPTER 15

How to Hit on a Girl in the Gym

These days, the gym is the social center of your world.

The gym is like the back of the bus in eighth grade—a cauldron of hormones and blood flow. Everywhere you turn, there are hot girls doing butt squats in yoga pants. What a time to be alive. Setting foot into the gym is like watching the preview thumbnail

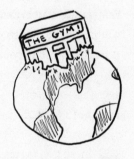

on Redtube.com—only the highlights. Now, I am straight drunk off horny juice, which is a mix of adrenaline, pump blood, and pre-workout.

When you get to the gym, your goal is to conquer the most death-defying lift in history—that is, until you spot a female gazelle grazing by herself around the free weights. You have been derailed, bro. At this point in your lifting career, chicks can tell that you lift. Your confidence is at its peak, and you are ready to approach her. You may not know how to hit on a girl in the gym, but that does not matter because you are hitting on her just by being there.

Before we get into the approach, let's talk about the jungle for a second. Men, obviously we are lions; maybe even rhino-lions, yes, definitely rhino-lions.

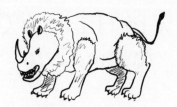

We are overly cocky, aggressive, all hyping each other up at the watering hole, aka the weight room, always looking for our next kill. And what do you know? Here comes the gazelle, aka a hot chick. Women are like gazelles, because they are beautiful skittish creatures that can run away from you really fast. They do not want to go to the watering hole, but they need that water to live. Now all you have to do is be there. Invite your boys, too; they will want to see this.

Here are a few tips on how to score that gazelle.

The Trick-Shot Mirror Checkout

Believe it or not, the mirrors in the gym also show the reflections of people besides yourself. Try standing in front of one and letting your eyes drift away from your own reflection. Do you see anything? Oh, what is that? A chick? Yes, yes it is.

The trick-shot mirror checkout is when you bounce your gaze off of, like, eight different mirrors just to check out a girl from across the gym. Do not be fooled, this is a two-way street. The rule is: If you see her eyes, she sees yours. Busted. You just got Chris Hansen-ed. Rookie. Go take a seat in the Smith machine.

Now, instead of transmitting your creepy vibes toward this inno-cent chick, you want to transmit your pump to her through these mir-rors. Let your gains do the talking. They are subtle, yet effective. There is nothing creepy about being shredded.

After you have given the trick-shot mirror a few attempts, you will quickly realize that she will always catch you checking her out like a creep, but she will never catch you with that glory swole. That is not going to stop you from trying. Every lion has to eat.

The Scenic Route

Sometimes in life, you choose the scenic route. In the gym, you are the scenic route. Make sure all the hot chicks get a glimpse. The scenic route is when you alter your entire workout just to lift next to a chick. Oh, you are doing leg extensions? Fuck that, looks like there is a dime hitting triceps on the cables. That is a green light for some pull-ups. Time your approach properly. Make sure she is resting while you are busy winning. Most important, make sure she catches that pump. Ide-ally, you want her to be so mesmerized by your rock swole that she approaches you. Maybe she will say something like, "Wow, I can't be-lieve you have such perfect form while lifting all that weight. Can you teach me? What are you doing after the gym? Do you want to come over?" Every single lift you've put up led to this moment. This is the definition of the glory swole.

The Mating Stance

In the jungle, a female lion always knows when the alpha male is ready to mate. That's the law of nature. The gym should be no different.

There is no single mating stance for the male lifter. This is a pose and an energy you have to discover for yourself through endless trial and error. As a guideline, though, every mating stance should have the shoulders back, chest out, chin up, and a constant arm flex. Similar to the ideal selfie pose, you want to look naturally swole. Everyone is different, so you will have to work a little to learn how to best broadcast your prized assets.

The Chase

Aka the only time I am going to fucking do cardio. The chase is when you post up next to a chick who is on the treadmill, coyly glance at her speed, and one-up her by at least 4 mph. By running faster than her, you are displaying that you are not only stronger, but also faster.

The chase is not a long-term game. We both know that you will not last more than six minutes on 7 mph so you need to make every moment count. Forget about easing into the sprint, jack that shit up and go. You are Nicolas Cage in *Gone in 60 Seconds*.

Once you have established your dominance and general betterness, meet her in the mirror and spark up some conversation. Ask her what she is training for, or if she wants to know what you are training for. Her answer doesn't matter, you are just letting her know that you recognize her dedication.

The Water Fountain

BRO TIP: Never pass up an opportunity to flex. Whenever you see a gazelle approaching the watering hole, drop whatever you are lifting and beat her to it. The water fountain is always a solid flex. Make it look like you are holding up the entire wall. She will be attracted to you because she will know how hard you are working based on your need for hydration.

The Drive-by

Take any chance you get to walk your pump past a chick. You think walking a dog gets a guy a lot of pussy? Try walking your pump. Walk straight past her, make no eye contact, flex like you just got out of prison. A well-executed drive-by will leave behind a trail of pheromones for her and she will think, "Wow, that dude smells huge." Jackpot.

The Muscle Counselor

You do not know much, but you know everything about fitness. Chicks love a knowledgeable man, so make sure your knowledge is known. If a chick is within reasonable proximity to you (if she is in the gym while you are), throw a bunch of unwanted advice her way. Women especially like this when their headphones are on. She looks at you and can only see some red-skinned dude flushed and overpumped moving his mouth when she is just trying to listen to *Serial*. You are none the wiser and continue speaking. She will eventually remove her headphones only to hear you during the tail end of your advice spewing something like, ". . . really get that ass tight."

Not to be the bearer of bad news, but if you are not a jacked black guy, then the Muscle Counselor ain't going to work for you.

—◍—◍—

The best part about my advice on hitting on a girl in the gym is that the entire time you will have barely said a word to her. We both know your voice isn't your best asset, unless it's grunting like a monster truck cuz of the three plates you just put up. Don't talk about it, be about it. And by "it" I mean those *gains*. Follow my tips and you'll be hitting back with your swolemate in no time.

CHAPTER 16

What Type of Fitness Chick Are You?

Newsflash, all you sexist pigs: It's the not the 1950s anymore. Women are bros, too. Among women's great achievements are: Beyoncé, the right to vote—and not just, like, for *American Idol*, but, like, for the American president, Ryan Seacrest—and baking; they are still pretty good at baking. Lastly, women have also achieved the right to bear arms, aka get a hard body. Fitness chicks are hot right now and forever, and if you happen to be a fitness chick, I am sure you love telling people about it. Luckily for humanity, I have developed a complex algorithm to identify which type of fitness chick you are. Proceed with caution, the results may be shocking.

Fitness Basic Bitch

Have you read the book *Skinny Bitch*?
  Have you recently become a vegetarian?
  Are you a vegetarian because you are against animal cruelty?
  Are you a vegetarian because a book told you it was healthy?
  Is that book *Skinny Bitch*?

At any point has your diet consisted of only liquids?

Are you recently single?

Is your entire fitness Instagram geared toward making your ex wish he never broke up with you?

Do you love posting pictures of yourself doing yoga in public places?

Is a big reason you work out so you have an excuse to post a selfie? #fitfam.

Are you currently choosing a filter for that mirror pic of you in your neon pink Nikes, wearing your sports bra over your regular bra and your Lululemons while showing a tasteful amount of camel toe?

Is your ultimate goal to have a thigh gap?

Do you constantly Instagram pictures of your gerbil food, which consists of three lentils, an avocado slice, and kale shavings?

Did you get this "recipe" from another fit chick's Instagram account?

Is she, like, totally your idol?

Do you weight train or strictly cardio?

Jk, are you running the Brooklyn Half?

Obviously you are, because you are a fitness basic bitch.

Bodybuilder Chick

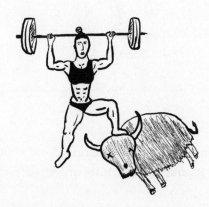

Have you changed your Instagram handle to include any of the following: "training," "fitness," "coach," "fit," or "body"?

When you wear clothes, does it look like your muscles are eating them?

Would others describe you as "annoyingly confident"?

Are dudes jealous of your capped shoulders?

Does it look like I can see the start of your vagina in your abs?

Does is look like you can strangle a yak with your legs?

Have you ever been asked if you have thought about competing?

Did the person who asked you about competing eventually become your trainer?

Was that an inspiring/eye-opening/humbling experience for you?

Do you fear anything anymore?

Can anything stop you?

Is that a quote you just posted on Instagram?

Yes?

Of course, because you are a bodybuilder chick.

Instagram Model

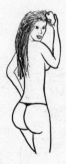

Do you like taking pictures of yourself?

Do you like posting these pictures of yourself for the approval of the Internet?

Do you like talking about yourself in the captions of the pictures you just posted?

Do an inappropriate amount of people follow you so they can see the moment you post your next picture, which looks exactly like the previous 3,467 pictures of yourself?

Have you somehow figured out a way to make this Instagram your fucking job?

Do you have an emoji check mark next to your name on your Instagram profile?

No way, so you are, like, totally verified?

Do you honestly think people read that *Iliad* of a caption you wrote when the reason they follow you is to try to count your bicycle spokes when you post a pic of yourself doing squats in a thong?

Do you inspire as many fap sessions as fit sessions?

Was porn your plan A?

Will it be your plan C?

Do I have a Google Alert set up for that? No doubt.

How many followers did it take for you to decide you are a model?

Have you ever worked at a Hooters?

Which nights?

Yo, which nights do you work?

Do I know every single detail of your body, but is your face more or less a mystery?

Have you suddenly become a personal trainer?

Have you ever met any of your clients personally?

When you say "training" do you mean "coaching"?

When you say "coaching" do you mean "selling chia seed recipes to basic bitches"?

Is Instagram your gym?

Do you really exist?

Are you the phone from *Her*?

No, you are an Instagram fitness model.

Squat Chick

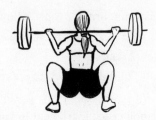

Would you say your butt is your best feature?

Did you used to be concerned about the size of your butt?

Are you now concerned about having to Pic Stitch all that ass into one Instagram?

Have you seriously considered auditioning for a rap video?

What is 2 Chainz like in real life?

Do you consider the big-butt craze to be your women's rights movement?

Do you consider squats to be your only movement?

Could I find this info on your Tinder profile?

Just to clarify, do you squat?

If you squat, but do not have a shirt that says you do, do you even lift?

Have you ever used the phrase "real men like curves, only dogs go for bones"?

Are you the girl warming up with some dude's max?

Do you have at least one picture of you squatting below parallel on your Instagram?

Do you have a cliché to describe everything in your life?

When you wear heels does it look like you should be playing a fife in a magical meadow?

To you a squat is which of the following: an exercise, an excuse to have a commandingly large ass, or the best thing to happen to thick girls since black dudes?

All the above, because you are a squat chick.

CrossFit Chick

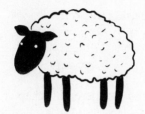

Is working out your new thing?

Is this something people know about you?

Is this the only thing people know about you?

How many times a day do you remind them?

Without social media posts, would people have any way of drawing the conclusion that you work out?

Did you give in to peer pressure easily as a child?

Which one of these animals describes you best: a sheep, a lemming, or two sheep?

How many rounds did you complete? *wink*

Do facts make you defensive?

Whoa, whoa, whoa, just asking.

I probably just went to a bad gym, right?

Are you all of a sudden gung-ho about working out?

Prior to that, which of the following would best describe your level of exercise: wishful, nonexistent, or fictional?

Did you see results when you started?

That's great! Have you seen any since?

But you *feel* better, right?

Are you still with the dude you lost your virginity to?

So you have had sex with other people?

Would you say it was better than the first?

So you admit the first thing you try is not always the best, right?

But you swore he was the one, didn't you?

But he let you down, didn't he?
Did he break his promises and leave you damaged?
How are you not getting this yet?
You are a CrossFit chick.

So to all the muscle bros out there, this chapter is meant to learn you on all the types of fitness chicks out there, walkin' all sexy-like around the weight room. The gym is no longer a meat locker, so step up your game. Fitness chicks are here to stay and if you want a shot at landing these lovely ladies, you better be in the gym getting those gains.

CHAPTER 17

One-Night Stands

You have been hitting the gym seven days a week for almost a year. Take a minute and try to think about what your life was like before you set foot in the Iron Throne. It's tough, right? Do you remember that you used to have a social life outside of the gym? Do you remember that you hung out with chicks who were not as obsessed with the gym as you? Believe it or not, life outside of the gym carried on while you locked yourself in the boneyard hitting news PRs on the daily. I bet some of those chicks even remember who you are. And if they didn't, they will now. It is officially time to take your swole outside the gym and apply those gains in the real world—aka, get some pussy.

Here's how it goes down. It's Friday evening, you just wrapped up a swole sesh, and you feel alive. You crushed a triple-scoop protein shake in the locker room and your phone buzzes. Oh shit, fresh text alert. It's your boy and he demands that you get to his place for a pregame. Your mind races back to months before when you attended your last pregame. You remember that feeling, and you want it back. Go get it.

You pull up to the pregame and something just feels right. It's one of those nights where you feel it in the air: You are coming home with the prize. That being said, you decide to pregame appropriately and get drunk to be interesting, but not wasted to the point of no boner.

After a sufficient pregame with you and seven of your best bros, you rip over to the bar. Fridays at the Tavern. Cheap $1.50 well drinks and 50 cent Bud Lights. You buy the first round of twenty Bud Lights because it is your night. No tip. For some reason the alcohol hits you harder than it did before, which startles you because you are bigger than you were before. Fuck that, you are invincible. Make a few more toasts with your crew and get the night started.

Whoa, you feel strong. You exhausted all your conversation topics with the crew during the pregame and can't stand around looking at your cell phone much longer. It is time to talk to a chick. It just so happens that your usual chick squad just walked in with a new addition. There is a target on her head and best of all: She does not go to your college. Awesome. Time to bombard her with generic statements about your school and your workout split and call it a conversation. And since she is visiting her friend, she has a free pass to bang whoever and not be called a slut. This is straight diplomatic immunity.

As you two talk, do not think of the conversation as flirting— think of it as running down the fucking shot clock. You are filling in the space between sips of her drink and, to your surprise, the exchange is going pretty well. Want to know why? Because you lift.

After fifteen minutes of conversing, you can tell your window to make a move is closing rapidly. Any second now, one of your boys is going to come shove you out of the way. Take advantage of the loud-ass music blaring and use the opportunity to whisper something non-threatening in her ear, but make sure your body language says otherwise. You are an alpha. Bingo.

After there is some sort of mutual touching, you have reached your first major checkpoint in the night. Now pull over the fucking car because you are not moving for the rest of the night. The moment a chick touches you she is telling you with her body what she can't with words.

I do not care if you are clenching ten Bud Lights in your bladder. You are not moving. I don't care if your boys are dead. This is your night.

Oh shit, what is this? She's holding your hand? Jackpot. Once you get that hand hold, you know it is on. Be wary, though. The hand hold immediately triggers her friends' instinct to cock block. D up and box them out. You see more of them. They are coming in hot like a pack of hyenas. You have two choices: Kill them with kindness or with shots. Whichever comes first.

Okay, you are in the clear, for now. Her friends like you, and they're all super drunk from the four kamikaze rounds you bought. Now your bros are moving in on them. Well done. You are the maestro. Time to bring her to the dance floor. It doesn't matter if Lynyrd Skynyrd is playing. Get her to that floor and slowly touch foreheads then start making out. You got this, bro.

You did it. Your mouths are like car-wash-strength vacuum cleaners running on $500 worth of quarters. Relish this moment while you can, because any minute now she is going to dart to the bathroom with no warning whatsoever. This is your make-or-break moment. You cannot lose this chick. You are shitfaced, but you are operating with unprecedented clarity and play out all the scenarios. If you lose her, her friends will swallow her up and she will immediately forget who you are. Find the girls' bathroom and wait close enough to it so that you can see her from a distance: #vantagepoint. As she exits, casually intercept her before she is touched by the crowd. Phew, success. This is the first and only marathon you have ever run and you are almost at the finish line.

Now it is time to refresh her memory. Immediately get back to more sloppy hooking up. Next thing you know you have a ton of bullshit pouring out of your mouth. You just whispered, "I want to spend the rest of my life with you tonight" in her ear. Bravo. You are making out and holding hands like you are in love. This could be it.

Nope. From a few feet away you hear, "Becky, we're leaving." And then everything freezes. You stare at her dead in the eyes and she says, "I think I am going to stay." Your dick spits out a little pre-cum. Don't worry, those are your dick's happy tears.

You are both free now. Free to continue hooking up like primates trying to save humanity. You both have been here way too long and are way too drunk. It is time to go. You know this because you puked in the bathroom at least once and the lights are on.

There is no discussion of, "Let's go back to my place." You walk out of the bar holding hands and somehow end up in an Uber SUV to your apartment. Just be happy you got there in one piece, do not question how. It is magic. Now what do you do? You guessed it, fix her up a nice cocktail to show her that you are an adult. "You want a mimosa?," aka leftover André from New Year's and your roommate's OJ with lots of pulp. You are a couple sips away from the spins so you head to the bathroom to warm up. Give yourself a pep talk before the game. Walk out of there with drunk, seductive eyes and start making out again.

It is time to head to your bedroom. Go straight to your bed because that is your only move and your only piece of furniture. Test the waters a little bit. Feel her waist, cop a titty feel, all good there. Go time. You undress her first without thinking. Next thing you know she is in her thong and you are in your jeans with your belt still on. Commence dry humping. This is the moment your boner decides to come alive, almost too much so. Pace yourself, bro. Roll her over and start finger blasting her. Go into the shed and bust out the lawn mower while her panties are on. That is a little move I learned from a YouJizz .com video my boy Matty showed me back in the day. You know the one I am talking about.

You finish finger blasting her and your dick has yet to be touched. Whatever, this is about endurance. Take off her thong and go down on her, Magellan. Take this opportunity to take off your jeans and start jerking off on the side of the bed. Who said guys are not good at multitasking? This is like running the engine room of the *Titanic* by yourself. You are not sure about this whole eye contact thing and think it might be sexy to establish eye contact. You link eyes and it is fucking disastrous. This is what a seal sees before it gets eaten by a killer whale. It is best to close your eyes and let nature take its course. Trust me.

Okay, now you have finally achieved your rock swole. It is super weak, though. You are one wrong breath away from pasta. Abort. Saddle up next to her and get that lawn mower going again in hopes that she reciprocates. You are a gentleman so you ask her to politely use her mouth. She obliges. Yes. It feels like the best blow job of your life and it is actually happening: #blessed. Careful now, make the right choice to cut it off early before you tap out.

The way things are going for you, you might as well put all your chips in. Roll her off you and tiptoe around her butt with your rawbone. She ain't having it. Denied. Gretzky wasn't talking about hockey when he said, "You miss 1,000 percent of the shots you don't take."

On to the main attraction. Grab a dusty Durex from your roommate's dresser. It is anyone's guess if it is expired or not. No time. Seems legit. Russian roulette. Your dick needs a vag sweater stat or you are going to be playing softball in a minute. Give her the juice. Straight missionary.

You have finally made it. Your pilgrimage. Be thankful that you are drunk because you are going all night. You mished her out for as long as you could. Your triceps are killing you but you got a sick pump. You caught some glimpses in the mirror. You caught yourself 'mirin'.

You have put in a ton of work, now it is her turn. Flip over so she is on top. You can see that she is getting close and this turns you on. But you cannot let her win this race. You have been nothing but disciplined the entire night and now it's time to let the dog loose. Grab her hips and drill her out like humanity depends on it. Finish first with seconds to spare, rip the conny off, toss it behind you: #BPoilspill. You don't care. You both pass out.

You wake up the next morning, and the air has a hint of regret and spermicide. The room smells like a tire fire. She leaps out of bed and tries to cover herself up as she gets dressed. You take this chance to make sure she is at least a 7. You meticulously study her body in the daylight: ass, tits, waist, face . . . you are good to go. Solid 8, bro.

Finish strong. Be a gentleman and walk her to the elevator. Give her a kiss on the cheek and a high five because you do not know what the fuck you are doing. As soon as those elevator doors shut, text the groupchat and exaggerate the hookup. "Got my d s'ed and my a l'ed. Gave her that A-Rod, g'ed her like I'm Derek." And then insert three fire emojis.

CHAPTER 18

How to Pack for Music Festivals

As many of you know from Facebook, music festivals are the place to get shithoused with your shirt off. Look in the mirror, bro. You're a lifter. Sirens should be going off in your brain. Visions of shirtless shuffling and going tongue deep in some Mollied-out yoga chick should be the only thing on your mind. Any opportunity you have to take your shirt off while double-fisting a couple of brews is an opportunity you will take. Though you can barely afford your gym membership, you will somehow come up with a way to spend $900 on a festival pass off StubHub. And, yo, if you are looking for tickets, hit me up. Uncle Dom's got you.

With a ticket in hand, you now have your pot of gold at the end of the rainbow. A reason to absolutely crush the gym for the next two months. Believe me, after a while it can get tough to hit the gym solely for yourself. Lifting to showcase your cuts for others is the true reason you lift. Hence why the music festival is so clutch. We are talking about three days of drugs, alcohol, dancing, drugs, sweating, alcohol, and zero food intake. This is either a recipe for shredded cheddar or a recipe for disaster. Either way, you win.

The key to music festivals is not to lose your swole after day one. Trust me, you do not want to come in looking like Tyrannosaurus flex and leave looking like Petri on an all-juice diet after a three-hour spin class. I've been hitting up music festivals since puberty. At thirteen I went with my mom to Florida for vacation, faked sick the first day, and hit up Ultra with a couple of dudes I met in the hotel. Been every year since, and then some. So believe me when I tell you that I am very much an expert. Let me be your guide to preparing for the three-day parking-lot-noise party/orgy that will change your life.

First up is packing. You are probably used to a huge gym bag filled with a bunch of tech and supplements, but a gym bag is not very practical for a music festival. What you need is the drawstring bag.

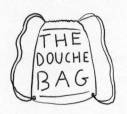

The drawstring bag is standard-issue bro gear. You are pretty much handed one as soon as you realize neon is the new pastel, which happens once you start lifting.

Drawstring bags are best for a few reasons. First of all, they are ideal to show off the body you've been working on all year long. It's simple clothes math, bro: Shirts were invented to pop the fuck off, and drawstrings were invented so you could accentuate that sick upside-down Christmas tree you've etched onto your back. You earned it, so show it off. Throw your shirt in your drawstring bag and prepare for the V. And by V I mean vag.

Drawstrings also solve the problem of what to do with your hands when you're not clutching iron. Since you will likely be shuffling or standing during the entire festival, the best position for your hands will be to have them clenched around the drawstrings. You may not know this, but you are unintentionally rocking one of the most prized poses in history: the flex rocker pose. By grabbing your drawstrings with your shirt off, you have that sick casual flex look going, with your biceps flexed, your lats spread, your chest out, and your traps un-trapped. Feels good, doesn't it?

Since you have limited space in your drawstring, you need to be smart about what you pack in it. The first item is life support, aka protein powder. Typically, protein is a pain in the ass to pack because it comes in huge containers that take up a lot of space. It is up to you to figure out how many servings you are going to need to hold you over throughout the entire music festival. WARNING: This involves high-level calculus. Whatever, we can figure it out with the power of Bro Science.

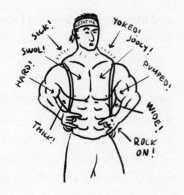

Okay, let's say you are at the festival for three days. Think about how many servings you are going to need per day for breakfast, lunch, and dinner. This equals three servings total. One serving equals two scoops, and a scoop is one thing. Now email all of these raw findings to NASA and await their reply.

I have their reply right here, actually.

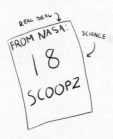

Based on NASA's findings, bring a small protein tub.

BRO TIP: Do not forget the scoop. How are you going to know how many servings you are consuming without the scoop? You're going to be rolling face so hard that you'll end up finishing the entire 5-pound tub. The scoop establishes order in your protein diet. Without the scoop you are shooting blanks in the dark.

In order to consume your protein, you need to pack a shaker cup. Make sure to bring the correct size—not too big, not too small, and without a bunch of gadgets like blender balls and shaker fences, because by the end of the festival, your unwashed shaker cup will have been baking in 100-degree weather inside your drawstring for three days. It is going to make Ebola look like a bowla Lucky Charms.

At this point, the only solid consumables in your drawstring are various pills. Not a bad problem to have, but you should probably have other forms of sustenance. Don't kid yourself, you aren't going to wait in line, lose your buzz, and pay $35 for a soft pretzel and a water at one of the food vendors. You did not come here to eat. The feeling of hunger is just a signal from your brain that your body needs nutrients, so you will need some dense mystery calories to feed your muscles, preferably in the form of putty. Reach into your drawstring and pull out whatever meal replacement bar you find, chew it, swallow, and keep raging. The last thing you need right now is to go catabolic.

BRO FACT: Contrary to popular belief, catabolic is not just a DJing cat, it is the death of your muscles and the end of the world as you know it.

BRONUS: Meal replacement bars are harder to chew than tire scraps, making them perfect to chew on while rolling face.

Next up we have the holy grail of Bro Science: pre-workout. Jesus' cup was literally filled with pre-workout during the Last Supper, and so should your drawstring bag be during the festival.

What is a meathead party stack without pre-workout? When I am raging, I don't just want my heart to beat inside my chest, I want it to grow inside of my chest. If Red Bull gives you wings, pre-workout will give you three wings, a missile launcher, and the ability to breathe fire.

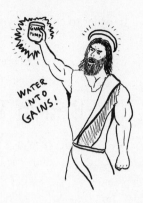

Thus far we have all the necessary ingredients to feed your body during the three-day bender. What about aesthetics? The most important and obvious reason you lift. Got you covered. Literally, covered. Covered in Pam. Pam is great to oil your muscles or use as a quick shot of essential fats in a pinch. Keep those t-levels up, which is Tiësto's remix of "Levels."

Lastly is gum. Be considerate, bro. You've been swagging down warm protein shakes and you are dehydrated from all the Molly. Nothing is worse than dry mouth and protein breath. No chick is going to make out with some dude whose breath smells like he just chewed on Iron Man's dick. Trust me.

There you have it. The essential music festival survival bag, or as I like to call it: The Douche Bag.

CHAPTER 19

Beach Weekend Pump Workout

Forget about Christmas, it's all about beach season, the official season of greatness. Beach season means that you are going to spend every single weekend at a tiki bar talking to other jacked dudes about how jacked you are, what your supplement stack consists of, and how you started drinking at 7:00 A.M. You count down the seconds until Friday so you can jump in your boy's Civic and rip down to the shore. And let's be real, bro. You aren't fooling anyone if you think you are going to hit the gym while you are at the beach. Not a fucking chance. If you are telling yourself that you are going to wake up hungover on Saturday at 1:00 P.M., spend a half hour at the beach so you can maximize your sick tan, and make it to the gym before two Bud Lights and a bottle of Fireball are waterfalled down your throat, you are a fucking liar. Since we are finally being honest, you know that Friday is your last day to squeeze every last drop of blood out of your heart into your muscles to prepare for the shirtless weekend around the corner.

It doesn't matter what muscles you hit during the days prior to the weekend—you are going to save or redo the most important muscles, aka the popcorn muscles, for this weekend-long all-you-can-pump buffet. Through decades of scientific animal testing, on myself, I have arrived at the perfect beach weekend pump workout. My workout is engineered around speed and efficiency and is guaranteed to give you that necessary glory swole that will be hotter than the sun and bigger than the ocean.

Workout Plan

BENCH

Not starting a full-body beach workout with bench is like starting a race and not flooring it when the flag is dropped. You don't do 0–60, you do 0–225. You're slamming down the accelerator, spinning the tires, and firing on all cylinders. Oh, what? You might blow out your engine? Good! Get out of the car and run the rest of the race using your arms.

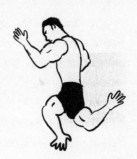

Every legendary workout begins with establishing momentum. Ain't no workout gonna get you going faster and harder than bench. Let's go.

SUPERSET! Immediately superset your bench with barbell 21s. Forget about the clips, too—ain't nobody got time for that. Chest and bis, it is practically one word. Chestandbis.

LAT PULLDOWN

Now I know what you are thinking: "But Dom! I can't even see my back. Why should I work it out?" I have three words for you: invisible lat syndrome. You need to pump your lats to create the ultimate illusion of size. If any haters ask, you will be able to tell them, "No, I actually cannot put my arms down, and yes I am actually this huge."

SUPERSET! Tricep pushdowns. Let's run through a basic equation: Everyone has a front and a back. The back of your body is 50 percent of your body. And your triceps are two-thirds of your arms. Therefore, your triceps are 116 percent of your body. Do the math. It is pretty fucking important. Get some pushdowns in and restore balance.

DUMBBELL SHOULDER PRESS/DUMBBELL SHRUG

> **BRO FACT:** Shoulders are an underrated body part because they aren't chest or arms. Understandable. But trust me, you should not neglect them. When you have your shirt off you look 300 percent bigger because of shoulder exposure. Your shoulders were created to pull your look together. Shoulders create separation and make you pop.

SUPERSET! Shrugs: Have you ever watched some porn and seen one of those dicks with the really big head and the tiny shaft? Ew. Do not let that be you. Do some shrugs. Pump up your neck shaft.

And there you have it. The perfect foundation for a total body pump. Now repeat this entire workout four times and you are good to go. Oh, shit. I forgot about abs . . . Crank out fifty slow and controlled crunches.

Okay, now we are all set. Just hang tight and wait for your ride to scoop you from the gym. Actually, since you are still in the gym, you might as well grab a few dumbbell curls and get that bicep pump rock hard.

Well, you can't just hit biceps without hitting triceps to even out your look. What are you, a rookie? Grab some more tricep pushdowns and call it a night. You've earned it.

Looks like your friend is here. Oh wow, you just realized you haven't hit forearms all week. He can wait. You need that forearm

T-shirt pump even though you will not have a shirt on all weekend. Rip out a few forearm curls.

You have come this far, so get some finger curls in, too.

Now check yourself out in the mirror one last time. Make sure your muscle universe is complete. Ah, good thing you are thorough, because it looks like you are losing your chest pump. Quick! Rep out some close-grip bench press. You just killed two birds with one fucking awesome exercise. Chest and triceps, keep it even.

Wait, how can you be even with just chest and triceps? You have to hit back and biceps while there is still time. Shove that dude off the pull-up bar and power through some close-grip underhand pull-ups.

Fuck, looks like your arms are too pumped now. How is this possible? This is awesome, but where did your shoulders go? Burn out some lateral raises and just run the entire rack.

SUPERSET! Superset every lateral raise set with traps.

Okay. You finally have the perfect beach weekend pump that will absolutely last until Sunday. All you need to do now is parade your muscle blimp around the beach. Everything is in proportion, finally. Beach daddy! Dap up everyone at the gym as you make your exit. You have to beat traffic. Peace.

Damnit. You were just about to leave and caught your reflection in the gym window . . . your abs are looking hella soft. Call up your boy and tell him you will be outside in fifteen . . . fifteen more sets. He will understand because he is your muscle friend.

Okay, you are finally in the car. Flex your bicep in the rearview mirror to check its status. Fuck. Looking soft, bro. Jump out of the car and get your ass back in the gym. Damnit, the door is locked. Gym is closed. No problem. Push-ups.

⚊⚌⚊

Moral of the story: No matter what you do, you will never be as big as your pump.

CHAPTER 20

How to Take Your Shirt Off

> **BRO FACT:** You lift to show off your body. Now, how do you expect me to show off when all that eye candy is covered by a shirt? There's no way you're going to catch me wearing a fucking body condom when it's 85 degrees outside.

Before you started lifting, you likely put on and removed your shirt without any thought. The simple act was not considered a major league spectator sport because there was nothing worth watching. Your life is different now. Taking your shirt off is not as easy as just *taking* your shirt off. Exposing your chest involves an intense level of strategy, hence the game: playing chest. There is an art to shirt removal. You want people to see your shirtless body, but do not want them to acknowledge that you are shirtless. You want it to seem like being raw bodied is your natural state. Like you came out of the womb and never put on a shirt. You want your shirtless body to tell the people to "Keep on moving, there is nothing to see here" . . . except everything.

Here is the Bro Science field manual on how to take your shirt off in some common situations.

The Beach

Jackpot. The beach is one of the few places where your shirt is expected to be off, so milk it. People go to the beach for two reasons: to sit around in a bathing suit, and to judge other people sitting around in bathing suits. The moment a new person sets foot on the sand, all eyes are on them. You are at the apex of getting attention. Capitalize on this moment to ensure that the maximum number of people are blessed by your sexually unbound upper half. It feels like you are getting Instagram likes in real life. What you want to do is locate your spot, drop your shit, survey the scene, and slowly circumcise your torso. Utilize the sunlight to highlight the cuts you don't actually have. Wow. Stay there. Hold that note. Feel that? That's not the heat of 102-degree sunlight, it's the heat from everyone's eyes on you. You just hooked them up with courtside seats to the show and they're getting horny. You just made their eyes pregnant. Nine months later they will be having vision babies of your body. Well done. Now jog into the water so you can repeat the arriving process, wet and shirtless.

At a BBQ

BBQ is French for lame outdoor party where no one's shirtless for some fuckin' reason. The trick to making it a party where shirts come off is to join or start up a physical activity. Immediately after the activity starts, let people know you're gonna pop your shirt off, cuz you're gonna work up a sweat. At any point after this, you can return to the party with your shirt on your shoulder, where it will remain for the rest of the party. You will now be the ripped hero instead of the dumbass who ripped his shirt off in the middle of an adult party . . . because no activity warrants being shirtless like cornhole.

A Pool Party Where No One's Swimming

First of all, this scenario doesn't make sense. It's like having a baby niece and not posting pics of you and her every holiday to harvest likes from chicks. What's the fucking point, you know? You've been here for two and a half grueling, fully clothed hours. You've been trying to spur some pool interest since the moment the FB event was created, but no one's biting. You already have a farmer's tan, the sun is setting, your window of opportunity is closing, and so are the legs of every girl who doesn't know what you are packing under that questionably patterned H&M button-down. You need to find a reason to get in that pool. Try some of the following methods: Make someone dare you to jump in. Try to push a girl into the pool in hopes that she'll push you back and you'll "fall" in. Be the tool who pretends he's going to jump in and then actually jump in. Lose a bet on purpose. If all else fails, be the drunk guy (my go-to move). Your shirt came off because you are shitfaced and jumped in the pool. Totally unplanned: #HardRockPoolParty.

At the Gym

What is the gym? Is it a dirty garage packed with sweaty dudes relocating iron? No . . . well, yes . . . but no, more than that, it's the one place you've always wanted to be shirtless. You're lifting, you got a pump, there are enough mirrors that you can see into the future. But thanks to whatever fucking Nazi came up with this rule, the closest we can get to being shirtless in the gym is wearing torso man thongs.

> **BRO TIP:** Secure a pump and pop your shirt off on your way out of the gym. As you're exiting, start up a meaningless conversation with the front desk guy. It doesn't matter what you talk about, just make sure you are fully flexed because you are now shirtless in the gym.

BRONUS: If your gym has one, use the outdoor/functional strength training area as an excuse to train shirtless, which is the only function of functional training.

At a Tailgate

A tailgate is a BBQ for assholes and sluts. That's how we do it in America. Everyone's drinking, getting rowdy, bro-ing out, and thinking, "How can I take my shirt off?" Do not be the first guy to take your shirt off or you will be swiftly and mercilessly branded with the scarlet *T*. *T* for "that dude." No one will even see your body because you will be wearing a thick turtleneck of shame. You don't wanna be the second guy either, because then you're just one of the two gay dudes with their shirts off together. You wanna be, like, the fourth guy with his shirt off a half hour later, after the first dude has been publicly dismembered and the other two have snuck off to dock in the back of your mom's Tahoe.

At a Party

This is a tricky one: You have booze on your side, but it's indoors and it's nighttime. Booze makes it okay to participate in what would normally be horrifying and regrettable acts: Pregging out a mutant, drowning a raccoon in a bathtub, and posting a flaccid dick pic to Instagram then pushing it to FB, to name a few, but somehow, you're still gonna be insecure about taking off your shirt. The key is to make being shirtless the thing to do. Start a dance party. Get into a flex-off. Start a fight. Play strip drinking games. Or just preface the night by cautioning people that tequila makes your clothes come off. "Yo, fair warning, don't let me near the tequila, that's when my shirt comes off."

There is no point to lifting day in and day out if you do not plan on being shirtless as much as possible outside the gym. Utilize the steps in this chapter to make sure every shirtless minute is working for you, not against you.

CHAPTER 21

Gym Buddy Problems

Now that you are well versed in the various methods of attaining a gym buddy, you are going to start experiencing the usual problems that come with spending hours with someone every single day. See, a gym buddy is more than just a relationship. When you lift with someone, you are letting them into the most important part of your life. Let me learn you on the usual personalities you will encounter as you enter the market of gym buddies, and what you can do to make sure you don't end up sharing your finest hours with any of these offenders.

Tardy Tim, aka Skip Bailess

Tardy Tim is the dude who will text you and ask to lift at six, tell you he is on the way at seven, and then tell you he cannot make it until eight. This inconsiderate prick leaves you pacing around the gym, strung out on pre-workout, doing a two-hour warm-up. There is nothing worse than precisely timing your pre-workout and then sitting around with your thumb up your ass waiting for your gym buddy no show. This is like facing a fistful of Viagra only to have your booty call tell you she is tired and cannot make it, leaving you with a feature-length boner while you're in bed listening to the Weeknd CD you teed up. I just rearranged my entire schedule so I could lift with you. If I wanted someone to make me a promise and not keep it, I would just call my dad. For real, bro.

Slippery Steve

Slippery Steve is somehow *never* lifting the same body part as you. It is easier to schedule a meeting with Manti Te'o's girlfriend in Atlantis while solving a Rubik's Cube and riding a chupacabra than it is to schedule a workout with this salamander. The only body part you can lift today is the exact body part he did last night. And the only other lift that both of you need to hit is legs, and fuck that. You try your best to reason with this guy, but it's pointless. Like, if we are trying to figure out a workout split and I say I need to hit chest, and he needs to hit back, I should win because I need a spot for chest day. He does not need a spot for back. He does not even need to lift his back. Chances are that if you have a Slippery Steve as a gym buddy, you aren't getting any buddy lifts in at all.

Half-assed Howie

If you typically do four sets, Half-assed Howie does three. If you do five exercises he does four. Case in point: It is arm day and this is the guy who will say you barely need to hit your arms because you hit them on chest and back day anyway, then he pops out nine total sets and leaves. Do you even lift, bro? The Half-assed Howies of the world love to spread bullshit. They are like that chick who cannot stop posting Elite Daily articles on Facebook about what she needs to be doing in her twenties. Half-assed Howie will believe anything he reads. Like that one interview with some amateur bodybuilder who claims he barely works out his arms and now has thirteen-inch cannons. This is a downward spiral into CrossFit, trust me. Anyone like Half-assed

Howie is not your real friend. He is the first guy to sound the "over-training alarm" to justify his bullshit thirty-minute workouts. Listen, it is not overtraining. It is *overgaining*. I am trying to go HAM, and you are giving me straight bologna, bro.

Pushy Paul, aka Cardio Cal

This dude always wants to do cardio, aka steal my gains. He is out to get you; someone call the cops. This is the same guy who actually counts his macros. Cardio Cal is all shredded and pushing you to be better and shit. Fuck this guy. Telling me not to drink too much and to watch my diet. Why do you care so much, bro? This guy loves his Lululemon tech gear and the newest Nike runners. He comes to the gym looking like a neon advertisement for big fitness brands and will not stop trying to convince you to run this year's marathon every time he sees you in the locker room. Worst of all is the fact that this guy will actually get you to feel bad about not doing any cardio. Do not be sidetracked by this impostor. Keep your eyes on the prize (your biceps).

Headphones Hank

Headphones Hank is not a bad dude, he just cannot lift without house music blasting in his ear from his noise-canceling headphones. I do not need to listen to Hardwell's new podcast during my set. Half the reason I have a gym buddy is to vent about my shit and talk about getting box. If you are going to have your headphones on I may as well lift with nobody. At this rate, you are just a guy that is working in with me. Lifting with your gym buddy while he has his headphones on is like getting a hand job from an ex-girlfriend. Yeah, I am going to finish, but I did not really need you here for this in the first place, and you were my last resort anyway.

Phony Phil

Lifting with your gym buddy is like being on a date. Your focus should be completely on me. I am holding hundreds of pounds over my chest, and you are pretending like you got me, bro, with your phone in one hand and your dick in the other. Literally, what the fuck on earth could be more important than this lift right now? What is happening on your phone that needs your attention more than me? I could die, bro. Or even worse, you could miss out on this sweet set I am about to do. It's dangerous. It's sexy. It's sexy because it is dangerous. And you are missing it. I hate you.

Now that you are progressing through the evolution of the lifting man, don't forget that there was a time when you were a skinny noob hunting for a gym buddy and may have even been one of the culprits above. Times have changed. Now you're the dude walking around the gym like an alpha god drawing lesser planets into your orbit. You now know exactly what to look for to ensure your swoldier battalion is stacked with gains: #fireARMS.

CHAPTER 22

There Will Be Grunts

Just like breathing, grunting is in our nature. Grunting was the first language, followed shortly after by emojis.

Grunting is simple: Grunting equals force. There have been thorough studies by Bro Scientists worldwide proving the undeniable fact that grunting is a sound. And as science is well aware, the bigger the sound, the stronger the object. For example, house music. When you're at any music festival, rolling face, the house music tent will pull you in by the sheer power of sound. Embrace it.

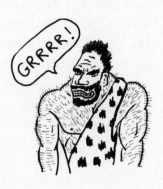

Your grunt explains who you are. It is your identity in the gym. Your grunt is your handshake. Your grunt says, "Nice to meet ya, I am going to be lifting enough weight to fuck your head off. You do not want to miss this."

Listen, telling me not to grunt in the gym is like telling a shark not to be awesome. But just as with beating off, there are times when it is appropriate and when it is inappropriate to grunt. As much as I want to, you are not going to catch me fappin' it while I am in the buffet line at Sizzler. And you are sure as shit not going to catch me grunting while I am lying on my stomach doing hamstring curls.

So, here's the deal: Grunting is reserved for weight that is impossible to be moved silently. If you're in the corner pushing baby weight, I better not be hearing you. It's bad enough I have to see you. You want to make a lot of noise and get nothing done? Go join a protest. Now here are some examples of the types of grunts you will encounter in any Iron Throne.

The Generic Single Grunt

The single grunt is like a shotgun. It is standard issue. It is loud and it is powerful, but you are not going to draw too much attention to yourself. The single grunt typically releases itself during low-rep heavyweight exercises like deadlifts and squats.

The Long Extended Hiss

What are you, a deflated kiddie pool? You belong in a backyard entertaining children, not in this gym. You are not even a real pool. You are the lowest type of pool. You cannot even retain fucking water. With each rep you are slowly deflating. Sitting there collecting mold between your stagnant muscles. Congratulations. You managed to fuck up breathing.

The Short Hiss Burst, aka the Bitch Hiss

Good stuff, hoss. You are now a deer. This is the noise that deer make when they are trying to sound threatening, but trust me, there is nothing threatening about your skinny head and shitty body resting on four Popsicle sticks. Deer are here for three reasons: to eat salad, to get shot, and to dent my Civic. I swerve into deer, bro. By letting out the bitch hiss, you are signaling to all the real lifters in the gym that you are not one of us. Do us all a favor, including yourself, and keep that embarrassingly weak sound to a minimum.

The Loud Extended Yell

You are louder than an eighteen-wheeler. Usually four wheels are enough to support most people, but you need fourteen more because you are fucking huge. At this point, your body is as wide as it is tall and you look like you came attached to the deadlift platform.

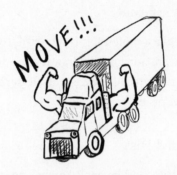

The combination of all the plates stacked onto the bar, your Juggernaut aesthetic, and the grunt you emit makes other lifters steer clear of you, because you scare them. You want everyone in the gym to see you and you do not care who you piss off. As far as you are concerned, you are the only one on the road. You only share the road because they do not make roads big enough for you. Basically, you should only let out the loud extended yell if you are a beast. You will know when the time is right because the weight you lift will not be possible to lift without the added pressure of the loud extended yell.

The Long Growl

No surprises here. You are a bear and your lift is genuine struggle. You are misunderstood. You could maul a child or be doing tree pull-ups, but either way you are here to do work. You are so big that people have been looking at you like you are out of place no matter where you go. You love it, because this is your land and everyone else is just hiking through it. You are not trying to draw attention to yourself, but you are, because every time you grunt, the entire gym shakes: 45lb plates fall off barbells. Mirrors explode. Even the smoothie girl gets a little wet. You don't care. You are busy getting huge and scaring the shit out of people.

So, there you have it. When it comes to your grunt, make sure you choose the right one. The best rule of thumb in the boneyard is not to force your grunt. If you have to try, then it is not real. Once you start putting up daddy weight, your grunt will find you. Eventually you will be grunting so much that you will forget how to speak in words. Awesome.

CHAPTER 23

Look Big, Get Big

Whoever said, "It's what's on the inside that counts" never set foot in the gym. You lift so you look good on the outside, which will make you feel good on the inside. So focus on what's important and double up on your look by making sure your gym gear is on point. You want your gym attire to make you look bigger than you are because if you look big you will get big. Simple math. Here is how.

Shirts are key. Shirts are the lead singer. They are Adam Levine and the rest of your outfit is Maroon 5. We both know everyone is only looking at your upper body anyway, so dress it right.

Now, the type of shirt you wear to the gym depends on which body part you are training that day. Ideally, you want to build up to wearing a tank every single day. My gym is like Tiananmen Square. I'm bringing the tanks. But you need to earn that right and, until you do, follow the guidelines below to maximize your gain gear.

Chest

You want to wear a tank on chest day so you can get that upper chest cleavage going on. If you do rock a tank on chest day, you better make sure your chest is shredded. You want your audience to see chest stria-tions, not man tits that look like water balloons.

On chest day you can also get away with a really tight T-shirt to sculpt that chest out. Be careful, though. The last issue you want to run into with a tight T-shirt is wearing one that is too small and makes you look like you are trying too hard. Rest assured that you will eventually find that perfectly fitted T-shirt, and you will *buy it in bulk*. Do not be disappointed when you realize you have spent $2,000 over four years on packs of T-shirts and wife-beaters that do not fit you properly. It is worth the expense to find that one T-shirt that fits you perfectly. You will find yourself wearing this T-shirt at the gym and at every single social event outside of the gym. It's an invest-ment, bro.

Back

The back is tricky because it is hard to tell if you have a back pump or not. As a gym bro, you probably want to wear a T-shirt on back day. Chances are you have some pretty wide lats at this point and your back is starting to resemble a turtle shell or a filleted fish. This means that you are ready to rock a tank or, better yet, a stringer. Go ahead, rock that back thong like Apollo Creed.

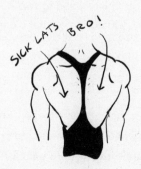

Legs

On leg day, you wear a long-sleeve T-shirt. Roll up the sleeves to expose those forearms and hide the fact that the blood is being robbed from your arms and going to your legs. The long-sleeve shirt being clenched around your forearm will make your arms look bigger even though you are not lifting arms at all. The perfect crime.

Shoulders

No matter what stage of the evolution you are in, you are going to look forward to shoulder day. Shoulder day is mandatory tank day. It does not matter how skinny you are; bust out those shoulders, because at some point during your lift, you will look shredded. Not wearing a tank on shoulder day is like not responding to the 2:00 A.M. "You up?" text. Take advantage of this. Shoulder day might be your only day of the week to look diesel.

Now, instead of a tank, you might choose to rock a cutoff on shoulder day and that is totally cool.

> **BRO TIP:** If you are going to wear a cutoff shirt, then wear a fucking cutoff shirt. Do not wear a beater under it. Wearing a beater under a cutoff is like wearing two condoms. You only need one. And really, you don't even need one.

Arms

Aka No Doubt Day because either way you are going to get a sick pump, no doubt. Wear whatever you want. Arm day is freedom. Arm day is what America stands for. Want to wear a T-shirt that is two sizes too big? Go ahead. Your arms are going to stretch those sleeves out by the end of your workout. Thinking about rocking a new tank that you aren't sure about? Today is the day. Fuck it, do not even show up to the gym with a shirt. No one is going to get in your way. Bis and tris. Buy yourself a steak dinner. Try to stop me.

So what are you waiting for? Get your ass into the gym and get that glory swole.

CHAPTER 24

What Your Gym Gear Says About You

When it comes to lifting, all that is required is you and gravity. Though lifting is the most basic of activities, you never want to look like a basic bitch, so you gotta dump a bunch of hard-earned cash into your gear. Remember, the gym gear that you choose will determine the type of lifter you are going to be. Choose wisely.

Gloves

Maybe you are lifting and you are thinking to yourself, "Ouch, these rugged iron weights are hurting my frail, velvety hand skin. Maybe I should start wearing lifting gloves so I can continue to give my boyfriend hand jobs with my buttery man paws." In that case, lifting gloves are for you. But if you want to feel what it's like to grab thunder and arm wrestle Zeus, then lose the gloves, earn your calluses, and contribute to the historic skin medley that collects on the knurling of the barbell. This is your heritage. This is your Ellis Island. Get hard, go raw: #RawNation #RawnaldReagan #RawmenNoodles #Rawmageddon #Rawesome.

Wrist Wraps

Wrist wraps are like spoilers on a car. Yeah, you are probably going to need a spoiler if you are driving a Formula One race car, just like you might need some wrist support if you are power cleaning 315lbs, which you are not. You do not need a big-ass wing on your fucking Mitsubishi Lancer just to drive to the mall, and you are not going to need wrist wraps to dumbbell curl 35lbs. But wrist wraps will make your forearms look bigger and spoilers will make your dick bigger. I highly recommend them both.

Toe Shoes

Shoes serve two purposes: to protect your feet and to protect others, so no one has to look at your fucking toes. But toe shoes? Wearing toe shoes is like wearing pants that have a specific sleeve for your dick to fit into. I did not ask for this fucking eye poison. Do you really think having your toes move individually is giving you the edge? How about you just lift harder and stop creeping everybody out with your toe cocks. You look like some sort of amphibious douche ninja. Give it a rest.

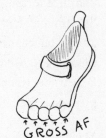

GROSS AF

Lifting Belt

You wear a lifting belt for support on heavy exercises, like squat or deadlift, and that is cool. But if you walk around the gym with a lifting belt all of the time, 95 percent of the time you are a fat dude. Or you are old. There are things that you simply do not need back support for.

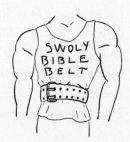

SWOLY
BIBLE
BELT

Bitching to your other over-the-hill friends about your nagging wife while aimlessly ambling around the gym is one of them. If you spent more time actually working on your lower back than you did walking around with a belt on, you might not need a belt anymore. But what the fuck do I know . . .

Joint Wraps/Compression Slips

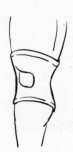

If you are wearing a knee brace, then you probably got busted up doing cardio. But are your limbs literally going to fall off if you do not have these weird joint wraps holding them together? That is what I thought. Lose the wraps.

Compression Clothing

The dude rocking compression clothing thinks he is an athlete because he is training for his intramural work basketball league. He might be an athlete, but chances are he is not, because if he were, he would not be at this gym. He would be on a fucking basketball court actually training. Why would you need to wear leggings under shorts in a heated fucking gym other than to look like you are training harder than you are?

Fitted/Snapback Hat

If you are wearing a snapback hat to the gym, then you used to be the guy wearing a fitted hat. You are a tool in all circles in and out of the gym. The fitted hat is like tagging wild animals. I am all about looking good in the gym, but if this extends into headwear you need to rethink some shit. You are not going to be working your ass off in the gym if you are too busy trying not to break a sweat in your limited-edition Yankees fitted with the stickers still on.

Headbands

Unless you are me, do not wear a headband. I wear headbands because I am anabolic. I marinate my headbands in pre-workout and cut a nice slit into my forehead. Goes straight to my brain. #MuscleBrain.

Elevation Training Mask

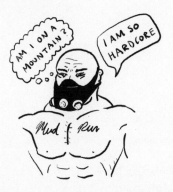

You are almost as bad as the dude wearing toe shoes. For $80 a pop, elevation training masks will restrict your oxygen so it feels like you're training on a mountain, and it simulates breathing through a fucking straw. Now have you also asked yourself, "How can I look like an asshole faster and more decisively than ever?" With this mask, you'll no longer have to waste time irritating people with your personality and conversations about Tough Mudders. Now they'll just know you're a tool from a distance.

The only saving grace of the elevation training mask is that you look like Bane. But you are not Bane. If you want to simulate high-altitude training so badly, just smoke weed between sets. You are setting foot into a gym and your concern is pulmonary resistance and strengthening your diaphragm? Go sign up for your next mud run and let me lift this fucking weight.

No matter what fitness apparel trend you are currently into, just know that it will change in, like, two months. Eventually your entire wardrobe will consist of only fitness clothing, most of which you will never wear again, and you'll forget what you looked like in a pair of jeans. This is a good sign.

STAGE 4

Gym Bro

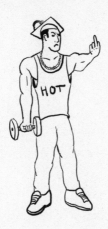

Bro, you are fucking crushing it. At this stage, you actually have some experience and knowledge under your lifting belt. You have pushed past your first plateau and you get some stares when you enter any gym. You are rocking tanks every day, including leg day, and a stringer on back day. You subscribe to *Muscle & Fitness* magazine and your homepage is Bodybuilding.com. And your Incognito homepage is Redtube .com. Congratulations! You are a true student of Bro Science. Your aesthetic physique is good and you peaced your girl because you realized you're prettier than she is . . . but deep down, you know you're not pretty enough. Your chest could use some work for sure . . . triceps, too . . . Actually your back could be wider. Quads . . . where are they? Biceps could be bigger, of course. Shoulders are looking flat; traps, too . . . What happened to you, bro? Do you even lift? Ah, fuck, you're small.

CHAPTER 25

How to Skip Leg Day

Every true Bro Scientist knows that working on legs is the fucking worst. Leg day takes all the motivation in the world, it fucking hurts, and legs aren't arms, or chest . . . or shoulders . . . they're not even back.

Last week you promised yourself and your gym buddy that you were gonna destroy legs this week, but like the true curl bro that you are, you're lookin' to do a workout without the work. Respect. You've come to the right place. Here are the Brofessor's foolproof ways to skip leg day guilt-free.

Phantom Injuries

When it comes to lifting, no minor injury or discomfort should be ignored. At this point, you've had a few minor real injuries that you chose to ignore and that resulted in weeks out of the gym. You know better now. The last thing you need is to see a doctor who tells you not to work out for the next six months. Once that happens, you know you'll end up shoving Domino's down your throat and binging Food Network reality shows while your mom yells at you to get a fucking job. However, on leg day, injuries are a different story.

Remember that time you checked your phone ten times in an hour because you swore you felt it vibrate ever since you got that chick's (fake) number at the bar last night? Apply the phantom texts to injuries whenever you feel a leg day coming on. As soon as you wake up on leg day, text your boy and let him know that you messed up your knee. You have no idea how, especially since you haven't used your legs since your last leg day, which was your first leg day, and your last leg day. Something's up, though. Your body is telling you not to risk hitting legs today. Listen to it.

Now, just because "your knee is definitely very fucked up," you aren't about to skip the gym altogether and lose all your gains. The best way to recover from this phantom knee pain is with some heavy, sloppy-form cheat curls.

The Feeling Ain't Right

For you to successfully complete a leg workout, the entire universe needs to be aligned. If you can convince yourself that even one little thing is off, it's best not to force a leg day.

Let's say you sprint to the squat rack fully loaded on pre-workout and ready to set a new PR, but you check your phone real quick to see if you got any new likes on that selfie you posted in the locker room two minutes ago, and you realize you didn't include #swolepatrol . . . damn. That's your go-to hashie, how could you forget it? What's wrong with you? Is everything okay, bro? Maybe you should take a minute. You good? Okay, head back to the squat rack.

Okay. Go time. Load up a couple 45s and reconfigure yourself. Lift off! Wait, the bar feels weird. Fuck it. You're here to squat, so squat. Wow, you definitely felt off on your squat. Something ain't right. Put the bar back and check it out. Shit. You put a 35lb on there. Dude . . . get a grip. Do you need to see someone? So embarrassing. No one noticed, but you did. And that's one people too many. This day is not your day.

The Hunger Games

You get to the gym and realize you haven't consumed nearly enough calories to carry you through this one-man Iditarod. Your typical calorie consumption before workouts is more than enough, but if you're gonna lift legs, which is a big if, you're gonna go HAM, cuz a leg day needs to last you a month or two.

The plus side in this scenario is that you have conveniently consumed the perfect amount of calories to hit any body part other than legs, so you might as well do that. Waste not, want not.

Gone in Sixty Seconds

Since it's leg day, it takes you a while to build up the courage to get out of the house and into the gym. You've watched hours of YouTube bodybuilder clips, taken two naps to make sure you're fully rested, and eaten five bowls of rice to ensure you'll have enough energy to complete the workout. By the time you get to the gym, it's 6:00 P.M. and every single bro you know is there.

Turns out the squat rack and leg press are taken. Damn, what a bummer. This isn't your fault, bro. Don't even think about approaching the dudes who are using your equipment. Don't wait for a second. Don't ask how many sets they have cuz it's definitely a thousand. Fuck it. Ditch your entire leg workout. You didn't come here to stand around. You came here to lift legs, and you weren't even 100 percent about that.

Now you have a couple options: Either come back later and hit legs when the gym empties out or stay in the gym and hit arms. That's what I thought. You'll lift legs tomorrow . . .

Yawning

You just yawned once. There's no way you're finishing this leg workout. Go rest, bro.

The Priority Principle

You're all set up for leg day and catch a glimpse of yourself in the mirror and realize you don't have a pump. This is the saddest sight. You look like a hairless cat. So gross. If you've ever seen your arms without a pump, it's like you can't see anything else.

Don't worry, Uncle Dom has your way out. Apply the Priority Principle: Your arms look small today, but your legs look small every day. So which is more urgent? Bingo. This isn't an emergency. It's an *arm*ergency.

The Buddy System

It's leg day, so you hit up your gym buddy to see if he'll take the plunge with you. Turns out there's a reason he's your gym buddy in the first place: Because he ain't lifting legs today. He's hittin' chest. #Bros4Life.

You just beasted through a legendary chest workout yesterday, but you don't care. Your gym buddy needs you. Well, he didn't say that, but you know it's true. So drop everything and head straight to the bench.

Just like that, you managed to hold off on leg day guilt-free. Just make sure you get some squats in at some point, cuz you definitely don't want to be that dude with zero legs come shorts season.

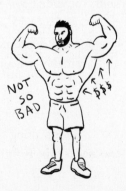

CHAPTER 26

What Is CrossFit?

By now you can tell how I feel about this bullshit fitness trend called CrossFit. Before one of the members of the Manson Family can talk your ear off about converting you to their lifestyle, let me save you some time and metaphorically punch them in the face with science. *Bro Science.*

First off, CrossFit is a class. I should just stop here. Taking fitness classes is like riding the bus. No matter where you want to go, you're not the one behind the wheel. You are crammed into a box with people who have no direction and are incapable of driving themselves. Are these the people you want to surround yourself with, bro?

CrossFit is great because you don't have to worry about exercising for a goal, because exercise is your goal. If you're trying to build the physique of what success looks like, then CrossFit is not for you. If you're looking to get really good at moving fast for an hour straight, then CrossFit is definitely your choice of fitness. The difference between lifting and CrossFit is the difference between building a house and being really good at aimlessly hammering nails into a board.

When it comes to CrossFit, the only thing you'll be building is cardiovascular endurance, or as I call it, "the ability to lose gains." CrossFit is intense athletic training for the professional non-athlete. This is good for sports like desk jockeying, running your mouth about how awesome CrossFit is, watercooler polo, and shot-putting a dick in your ass. Me? I'm always playing my sport. It's called walking around like a fucking beast. And living to fifty. Live large. Die large. Leave a giant coffin.

CrossFit is a lifestyle, so everyone tells me. Apparently, it's a lifestyle that starts in the gym and ends on your Facebook. CrossFit is so humble no one even knows you're in shape unless you post your workout. Me? I post one picture with my shirt off, and everyone thinks I'm an asshole. (Okay, two pictures. A day. No regrets.) There's nothing as infuriating as seeing one of these CrossFitters spamming my social media with videos of their CrossFit team "getting after it this A.M." Congratulations, you meet at least once a week with a bunch of other people led by some loon with no gains, and all you do is tell everyone about your experience. Bet you never thought you'd be twenty-four and in a cult.

CrossFit places a *huge* emphasis on form by taking complicated movements, getting rid of all that useless shit like effectiveness and safety, and replacing it with violence and danger.

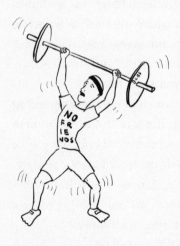

Case in point: the kipping pull-up. CrossFit has revolutionized fitness by teaching the correct way to do an incorrect pull-up. Groundbreaking stuff. Worst of all is that you're doing an entire workout incorrectly *for time*. Nothing like rushing through a workout doing movements you have no idea how to do. When you wake up with a couple popped discs in two years, don't worry, you'll look back on your CrossFit career and think how it was all worth it for that one day you finished first in your class.

If cheating your way through basic exercises isn't enough, you can also cheat yourself through weight with CrossFit. In CrossFit, everything looks like a 45lb plate, but don't be fooled by these fitness gypsies, that plate could be a ten pounder. CrossFit weight is the Spanx of weights.

Let Professor Dom break down the origin of bodybuilding. So, like one hundred years ago Zeus and Poseidon teamed up to create bodybuilding. Some humans have perfected the craft, like David, who's so rock swole he's literally a statue, and Arnold, who climaxes every time he completes a perfect bicep curl. These are the people that you should be emulating. Not some dude who's been saving up to hike Kilimanjaro in two years and orders a seltzer during happy hour. Whatever, you're a student of Bro Science, the largest school known to man, and the only way you lead is by example. Rest assured that one day there will be a CrossFitter who catches a glimpse of your glory pump after his class and will immediately approach the rack, grab a 35, and commence curling.

Respect, though. There are a handful of CrossFit dudes and chicks who are ripped up, but they're on ESPN (Saturday afternoons) flipping tractor tires and shit. They're the 1 percent. They know exactly how to perform each movement properly, because they probably lifted before they went over to the dark side. How else do you think they got that mass?

CrossFit goes against the very fiber of what bodybuilding is. In the gym, it's you vs. your reflection. No one else is gonna get your gains except you, and that's what makes lifting the ultimate competition. You have to make yourself get up every single day to lift arms, eat a ton of food, and deal with all the chicks who hit you up in the DM. It's a life not meant for many, but earned by few. If you don't like the sounds of it, then CrossFit might be right for you.

CHAPTER 27

How to Get Your Girlfriend to Start Lifting

Now that you are officially a gym bro, you are beginning to look for yourself in other women, because looking at yourself turns you the fuck on. You spend every moment at the gym perfecting every tiny detail of your body that no one will ever notice but you. The moment you get home, you shift your hypercritical gaze from yourself to your girlfriend. Great job. You are now transferring your borderline un-healthy obsession with yourself onto another human who never asked for it. What a lucky girl. Just like her Tri-Delta Grand Big, you are circling the body parts that she needs to work on, but with your mind instead of permanent marker. It's not your fault that you care about her so much that you expect absolute greatness.

With all that political bullshit aside, let me keep it one hundred thousand with you. It's all about dat ass. Dat ass that's so round and so firm that three dogs could bite into it and drag it into the woods . . . but there's still room for, like, one or two more dogs to sink into dat ass. That's what it's all about. Dat a$$. But your chick ain't gonna achieve that butt thunder by floating on the elliptical for ninety minutes while reading *Us Weekly*. You gotta make your momma proud and take your girl to church.

Here are some Bro Science theories on the best ways to get your girl to participate in the holiest of activities, lifting.

Bring Your Girl to Work Day

Tell her you want to spend more time with her and then pull the old bait and switch and drag her to the gym. In addition to great bonding time, it will be an excuse for her to try out those new yoga pants she just bought from Lululemon for $98 on your fuckin' credit card. Once she's in the Iron Throne she will see how much work you put into looking good for her . . . definitely for her, not just for yourself. When you get your swell on in front of a girl, you literally become a human boner right in front of her eyes. It's only a matter of time before she's hitting squats. This is called learning through osmosis. Girls get off on passion in men; guys get off on ass-in-dem-yoga-pants. It's not my fault. It's science.

The Power of Suggestion

Girls are good at two things: comparing themselves negatively to other girls and uh . . . I don't know, come back to me. Pass. When you catch your girl looking at an Instagram pic of a fit chick saying, "OMG, I wish I had her body," your first instinct is to grab her by the shoulders and say, "You can!" But guys like us . . . we're sensitive creatures, so resist this urge. Getting your girl to lift is all about very gentle psychological manipulation. It's a lot like doing anal. Try these helpful phrases instead: "You ever try lifting before? I think you might like it," or "Babe, you're way sexier than her. I'd love to show you off in the gym," and the old faithful, "Come on, come on, come on, just a little bit."

The Barter System

Make some sort of trade with her. Tell her you want her to do something you're into and then you'll do something she's into. Then once she starts lifting, back out of your end of the deal and tell her that she's really the one benefiting from this and make her feel guilty.

Motivation Is Key

For women, jealousy is the best motivator. I named my dog Jealousy because it's man's best friend. Subtly slip into the conversation how your boy's girlfriend lifts all the time and how awesome she is. This is the perfect crime. Your girl is too busy being jealous to remember that you're being an asshole. Congratulations, you have just entered your girl into a girl-on-girl race to be the hottest. No matter who wins, you win.

The Best Things in Life Are Free

Sign your girl up for a new gym that offers a free training session. Girls looove free shit. They also love attention from a neutral attractive guy that's not you. In one free session, this patsy will do all the hard work for you, like the infuriating process of explaining to a girl that lifting won't make her "bigger," and how the phrase "tone down" should only be used if she's asking too many questions during a movie. And she will listen to him because, again, he's not you. She now totally loves fitness. But be sure to pull her out before the trainer can spew any Euro training propaganda . . . and then give her a dose of Bro Science.

—◖▬◗—

As a gym bro, the only way you are going to commit to a long-lasting relationship is if your chick starts lifting. You are a lifter and when you think of the future, you aren't thinking about a bunch of kids running around at Grandma's house on Thanksgiving . . . gross. You're thinking about a chick who's going to wake you up at 6:00 A.M. with some dome then hit the forgotten muscles with you, prep meals with you during the week, and lift back with you at night. And lots of animalistic bonin'. Believe it or not, you can find this dream girl if you follow the tactics above. Make sure you tag me in all your #Swolemate Instagrams, which aren't annoying at all.

CHAPTER 28

Fitness Tips for Basic Chicks

Hello, ladies. Are you looking to achieve your fitness goals? Good, then this program is not for you. If you are skinny fat, no longer twenty-two, and want to be fit but don't want to do fitness, then I got the plan that will take the "work" out of "workout." You can nix the "out," too, since it's all done from home. So we are taking the "work" and the "out" out of "workout," and you're left with nothin', cuz there's nothin' to it.

Always Eat Breakfast

This is always the first rule of chick fitness. This is a much-needed re-minder to put food in your body when a new day starts. I know what you'll say, "Ugh, but I'm never hungry in the morning! Now I have to Seamless a $30 acai bowl. Metabolism, decisions, rules. It is hard being alive. And it's gotta be healthy, too? Ugh, do I even *want* to be alive? I don't know, what do you want to do? Literally kill me."

Worry not, you poor tortured soul, eating healthy doesn't have to be such a curse. It can also be a Tumblr picture. Posting a photo of healthy food has more fitness benefits than actually consuming those nutrients. This is because when you post pictures of healthy food people will think you are fit, and isn't that the point of fitness? If you just eat the food, how will anyone know how fit you are?

> **CHICK TIP:** Hoard random, exotic, hard-to-peel fruit from Whole Foods for $30 an ounce. Make sure it's brightly colored—bright colors equal fitness. That's why you look the most fit in your neon orange Lululemon sports bra. Notice Lululemon is also a fruit, and not a coincidence.

Fruit is great because you don't have to prepare it, you can just eat it. But what's more fun than eating? A twenty-five-year-old woman doing arts and crafts with her food. Grab a knife and spend the next ninety minutes hacking at your fruit, making pointless kaleidoscope arrangements for yourself, and your 295 followers. Then toss it in your fridge and "save it for later" or add wine and make sangria. Don't worry, you can just scoop the fruit out, since it gets all mushy and gross anyway.

At-Home Workouts

Scroll through your Facebook feed, and you'll find it's littered with fitness gold in the form of autoplaying fifteen-second at-home workout clips featuring a chick who looks like Ariana Grande, flopping around on the floor, scissoring the air, and doing butt kicks. These are the ideal workouts for someone who's tried working out and realized it's not for them. The best part about an at-home workout is you can do it anytime, like some other time.

Challenging Yourself

. . . is a good way to fail. Who wants to make things harder? People who want to experience the benefits of fitness? Ew. Challenging yourself is like using Waze to take you on the route with the most traffic. Why would you do that when you could just stay home? Instead, find things that reassure you what you're already doing is fine. Look for studies that "prove" you don't need to work as hard as you thought to get the results you're okay with. Look, here's a study that says drinking a bottle of wine a night is the exact same as committing to a well-regimented workout plan for an entire year. Good, that's what I was going to do anyway. I love fitness.

You're Not Fat, You're Bloated

Did you just spend four days in Vegas drinking booze slushies, eating buffet food, and railing Adderall so you don't sleep? Duh. Don't worry, you're not destroying your fitness progress, you're just bloated, that's all. Do a juice cleanse, detox, post a few motivational IG pics, and kiss that bloat good-bye. You just lost three pounds! Congrats! You are fitnessing. You're not slowly gaining weight because you're getting older and you drink all the time and eat shitty foods while your metabolism slowly grinds to a halt, you're just bloated.

Aim Lower

You will never look like the girl in the magazine; the girl in the magazine doesn't even look like the girl in the magazine. Don't try to achieve your dream body; you can't have that, it's not real, that's why it's called a dream body. Instead, try to achieve your real body, which is the one you already have. Congrats, you did it. Always love yourself, even if deep down you're not truly happy and want to change things for the better. Just say fuck it and have some wine. And if that doesn't work then just actually whine.

CHAPTER 29

Diets

Now that you're a gym bro, you're taking this shit seriously. Putting on mass has slowly evolved into a process that extends outside of the gym. When you first started lifting, the only thing on your mind was beginner gains. When you weren't in the gym, you were busy shoving whey protein and fast food down the hatch multiple times a day. Now that you're in your fourth year at UoBS (University of Bro Science), you've begun researching and taking notice of how bigger bros fuel up and cut down. Here's the quick-and-easy on the tried-and-true meathead diets, and some new trends that have popped up along the way.

Bulking and Cutting

Bulking is what you do during cold months when it's not socially acceptable to be ripping your shirt off in public. It's a time when you get to consume way more calories than you typically do in an effort to gain mass that you will eventually cut down once the warmer months arrive, while retaining muscle. Once you begin cutting, the goal is to shred the fat from your bulk and end up with more muscle mass than you had the year before. You want to pop your shirt off at the first beach day of the season and have strangers approach you to ask how you got so much mass while staying so lean. In theory, cutting and bulking should look like a yin-yang, but in reality, you're never not bulking.

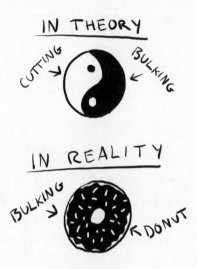

Eating Clean

Eating clean means to consume pure substances. The most popular of which is chicken. Just straight chicken. Throw in some steamed broccoli and you're in business. Eating only clean foods will come and go throughout your career as a lifter, because it gets fucking boring. Fast. As healthy as eating clean is for you, you have to eat a ton to put on mass.

Eating Dirty

When you start lifting, eating dirty will be preached by brofessors far and wide, and you will listen. Who in their right mind is going to say no to eating as much McDonald's as possible and then turn those filthy calories into muscle? You will see almost immediate beginner gains, which will jump-start your new life of mirror staring and macros counting.

Some lifters choose to continue eating dirty for life, but these dudes are usually so big that there aren't enough clean calories to feed their muscles in the world. They have no other options. If you're a bro, you might want to cut down on the fast food eventually. YouTube my video "Emergency Muscle Meals" for a breakdown on all the fast food used to get those gains.

If It Fits Your Macros (IIFYM)

IIFYM is a relatively new diet on the scene. Basically, you learn how to track the nutrients in everything you eat and make sure all of your total daily nutrients fit into your personal macros profile. IIFYM allows you to blend eating dirty and clean as long as they fit your macros. For a more detailed breakdown of IIFYM, turn to chapter 31.

What have we learned here? Just like anything else in fitness, you have options when it comes to your diet. Rest assured that no matter which diet you're doing at the moment, other lifters are going to tell you theirs is better, at which point you'll probably drop yours for theirs. What I'm saying is that you'll never consistently diet for more than three months at a time. As long as you end up in the gym every day, though, chances are you'll be fine. And if you run out of protein you can always hit up the McDonald's after your workout . . . it's an emergency, bro.

CHAPTER 30

How to Eat Chicken Without Wanting to Kill Yourself

You've started educating yourself on the benefits of not eating fast food five times per day and are in the middle of a clean-eating diet. You want nothing but pure protein feeding your muscles before and after your lifts, so you become more familiar with chicken breast than actual breasts. Oddly enough, chicken breast is among the least desirable of breasts, yet you keep on coming back for more. It may be the most boring of meats, but it's inexpensive, rich in protein, and easy to prepare. So you are going to fill your shopping cart with it and prepare it any way you can.

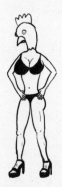

When it comes to chicken, there are only four types that are desirable: fried chicken, chicken wings, chicken parmesan, and chicken head.

But as a hard-core bodybuilder, you know these things are off limits, and for good reason. You can't go near any fried foods because you know you're never coming back from that binge. Chicken wings take too long to eat and you're never sure if you got enough protein from them, even after eating fifty atomic wings just to impress your Hooters waitress. You're not about to go home and get into the assembly line necessary to make a few chicken parm cutlets after spending two hours in the gym. And when it comes to chicken head, you're going to get as much as you can—but only on the weekends. Focus, bro.

So what are you left with? Your high and mighty ass is going to be eating bodybuilding chicken all day every day, which is closer to a Dr. Scholl's insert than it is to an actual piece of edible meat. It's a key part of the gym bro process. At first, it doesn't seem so bad. In fact, you spend the first few months loving bodybuilding chicken with some brown rice and salsa, making sure to Instagram it, #mealprep. But after three months of eating the same exact meal, you stare down at the piece of rubbery bicycle seat on your paper plate with your plastic utensils and your crushed soul and you think about quitting. But you'd rather kill yourself than lose your gains. That's why it's called a *die*t. So quitting is out of the question. Lucky for you, no one has to die here, uh . . . except for millions of chickens, that is.

Bear with me. Let's say one day you get married (yeah, see ya there), and you're stuck with one chick for, like, five years or however long people are married for . . . well, I can guarantee you ain't gonna be bonin' out your lady in the sports section of Wal-Mart like you did when you two first met. Chicken is like a married person's sex life. You need to mix it up so you don't lose interest. And there's no one better to learn you on chicken and sick positions than your Uncle Dom. But we're gonna stick to chicken this time. By the end of this chapter you'll be making chicken without wanting to kill yourself.

Prep

Fresh chicken keeps, what, max, like three days in the fridge? And you're going to be eating pounds of it over time, bro. So unless you wanna spend more time buying meat than being meat, you gotta buy in bulk. But that comes with its own downfalls. Anyone who has come back from the gym after blasting through a heavy-ass lift, hungry as fuck, knows that the worst part about cooking chicken is defrosting it. Trying to defrost a chicken in the microwave is more complicated than playing Minesweeper. You hit defrost and then input the nuclear launch codes required to melt ice, but even after seven and a half minutes of nonstop beeping, it's still rock hard in the center, so you toss it back in for another arbitrary amount of time. Now the edges are starting to cook and turn into bathtub caulk. So you got no choice but to take it out, and you're left with a half-microwaved, half-frozen chicken breast sitting in a pool of Ebola. You say fuck it and throw it on the pan anyway. The result is an overcooked Tempurpedic mattress that you have to eat or you'll go catabolic. Here's my advice: Avoid the defrosting stage at all costs. Go to Costco or BJ's or whatever place sells air conditioners in bulk and buy the thin-sliced "no-defrost" ten-pound bag of frozen chicken breast. This way you can just throw it all on the pan, no problem. It's like fucking without having to get a boner.

Taste

Chicken breast has no taste. In fact, saying chicken tastes bad would be giving chicken too much credit. Chicken is like that kid from high school that you spent four years sitting next to and the moment you graduate you forget his existence completely. The rare moment you eat anything other than chicken, you will momentarily be lifted to another place and forget all about that tasteless meat you've eaten three times a day since forever.

> **BRO TIP:** There's nothing you can do to chicken to make it taste good. You can only put things that taste good on it, and then eat the chicken as a consequence.

After years of trial and error, I give you Uncle Dom's Bodybuilder Hero Chicken Warrior breakdown. Follow my tips to trick yourself into forgetting that you're eating the equivalent of a deflated bicycle tire.

STEP ONE

Pretend the seasoning you added made a difference other than becoming the burned part you scrape off.

STEP TWO

Apply hot sauce. Hot sauce has no carbs or calories and sodium doesn't count as long as you don't read how much it has, so it's the perfect choice. Hot sauce is makeup; what's underneath is a reality you're not trying to face. And if you think you've got some outside-the-box, amazing recipe for chicken, then fuck off. Don't be that dude who thinks he's better than the chicken. You're not Bobby Flay. And even that dude drenches his chicken in chipotle.

Texture

Bodybuilding chicken isn't juicy, or well-marinated, or cooked under a brick for forty-five minutes. It's bird tits that you heat to get the poison out of for the sole purpose of making it edible in bulk quantities that you will reheat every day for the next week. You are gonna feel every single bite. You have to trick your brain into accepting as much dry, spongey chicken as possible before your jaw refuses to bite down on another piece. There are literally only two ways to do this.

STEP ONE

Shred the chicken. When you shred the chicken you weaken its primary defense: the amount of time it spends in your mouth.

STEP TWO

Chop the chicken into little tiny pieces and scatter it into whatever brown-rice-based side you've made. This is a speed move. This way you can shovel as much chicken as possible into your mouth before your brain realizes: a) that you're eating chicken, and b) that you fucking hate yourself.

Pairings

There's nothing your diet allows that is going to make chicken better. All your options are shitty, but you need something to mask the flavor. Here are some options to make the best out of your unfortunate situation.

VEGETABLES

There's an age-old debate in Bro Science about which food is worse: plain chicken breast or steamed broccoli. The true question is, are you eating the chicken to mask the veggies or are you eating the veggies to mask the chicken? This has yet to be answered and you shouldn't waste your time figuring it out. Let's be honest: You know you're going to buy vegetables and then let them sit in the bottom drawer of your fridge and rot. It's pointless to pretend otherwise. If you plan on pairing your chicken with vegetables, you might as well pair your chicken with air.

RICE

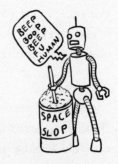

The blandest carb paired with the blandest meat. This is multiplying by zero. Rice looks like the gruel they would ration out on a space station after the earth dies.

The best thing about rice is that you can buy a rice cooker and cook that shit in bulk the same day as your chicken. When the chicken is done, chop it up into the tiniest pieces possible, mix it in with your fifteen pounds of rice, and take up your mom's entire fridge. Bam. Chicken and rice is the cleanest pairing you can get, so dig in.

POTATOES

If your first thought here was ooh, sweet potatoes, then you're an asshole. Sweet potatoes are the Equinox of potatoes. People who like them don't really know why they're good, but that doesn't stop them from telling you they're the best. Here's my message for these clowns: Get off your high horse and join the rest of the world, whose only concern is getting fucking huge. The only potatoes worth talking about are all-American, shaved-pussy-eating, V8-engine white potatoes . . . now we got ourselves a side. You know who eats white potatoes? People like Vin Diesel and The Rock. They say, "Fuck it, white potatoes are clean." I'd eat a lightbulb if it were paired with white potatoes, they're so delicious. WARNING: At a certain point, you are going to become obsessed with eating brown things like brown rice, brown bread, and brown potatoes, aka sweet potatoes. You're going to remain on that pedestal of "whole-wheat carbs" until you cross over into the Gym Bro stage, at which point you will only be concerned with consumption and the color white will enter back into your diet. This is your only real choice when it comes to pairings and not wanting to kill yourself.

SALAD

No.

—◫——◫—

If you've performed all these steps correctly, you will still hate chicken. Which brings me to the last step: Eat tuna. Have you ever had canned tuna? It's fucking awful. They say tuna is chicken of the sea, which means it's just as bad as chicken, but on top of that, it smells and tastes like whale pussy. Suddenly, chicken is not so bad. Now, I ain't no chef, but in Uncle Dom's kitchen I always got somethin' cooking. At the end of the day, your gains are fueled off food, and chicken is the premium-grade gasoline you want to run the engine. Eventually you're going to cycle through every possible chicken recipe known to man and start to see chicken as pure nutrients. You will find yourself literally shoveling tablespoons of chicken out of a Tupperware container into your mouth with no regard for taste. When this moment happens, look at yourself in a mirror and congratulate yourself. You have officially graduated from the Culinary Institute of Bro Science.

CHAPTER 31

What Is IIFYM?

IIFYM: If It Fits Your Macros. "It" meaning the food you're consuming and "macros" meaning the macronutrients that make up food, like protein, fat, and carbs.

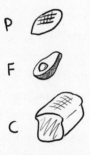

P

F

C

    For those of you who don't know, IIFYM is a form of dieting. Some not in the know are afraid to call it a diet, because they'll get reamed out by people who think a diet should only consist of salads and cardio. IIFYM goes even further than being just a diet. Just like lifting, IIFYM is a lifestyle. With IIFYM, you are free to eat whatever you want as long as you hit your protein, carbs, and fat requirements for the day. I'm serious, whatever you want. Double cheeseburger from McDonald's, ten-piece nuggets *and* a Frosty from Wendy's! Oh wait, still have room for a few Pringles at the end of the night? Of course you do. Because you're a macro-dieter and you DGAF.

The science behind macro dieting is explained with the phrase: A calorie is a calorie. This is great because I choose to live my life by repetitive, empty justifications: It is what it is, pussy is pussy, a calorie is a calorie. You don't need to tell me twice, you already did.

If you've been eating boiled chicken and reheated brown rice for every meal, hearing about IIFYM will get you wet. At this point of your Bro Science evolution, you've been lifting for half a decade and have everything you want: pussy, gains, and Instagram followers. What's the only thing missing here? Pop-Tarts.

So if you still find yourself "eating clean," aka on that chicken and rice game, then you're probably the guy still whipping together his Neknomination video after all the cool friends have been picked. Congrats, bro; you are the last friend. The rules of macro dieting state that your body can't tell the difference between carbs from brown rice and carbs from brownies. And now you're saying, "Oh, but Brofessor Dom, what about the glycemic index?!" What about it? I never understood it, and you don't have to pretend to, either. The only way to really eat clean is actually scrub your food with Windex . . . the glycemic Windex.

It's great for washing away the bullshit.

"Eating clean" is an outdated term and at one point was branded as Bro Science. There's some new Bro Science in town and it's IIFYM, which is also real science, aka Bro Science.

Now that you've heard all these promises about eating whatever you want, you may still have some questions. Understandable.

Trust me, when you first hear that you could eat whatever the fuck you wanted and still become a shredded gym warrior, you have your doubts. It's okay. Run with it. Give it a try. Get over the initial anxiety of trusting this so-called diet, and hit the Internet for some cold, hard research. Once you've handpicked specific articles supporting IIFYM, you should be ready to dive in. You're not. You need more. You're thinking that IIFYM is certainly gypsy magic and you will get fat if you try it. So you hit up the master on Facebook chat: your bro, who is a known macro dieter. He proves its credibility to you by showing you Instagram accounts of various bodybuilders who follow the IIFYM lifestyle. Your bro, who is bigger than you, sends you photographic evidence of some Freak Beasts who consume enough calories to feed a herd of yak, and really, that's all you need. This is foolproof evidence.

You're almost there. You got the tip in. There's no turning back, you're going in raw. After this, you'll go on a fact-finding mission— *Muscle & Fitness*, Bodybuilding.com forums, and iifym.com, which looks like the least credible site ever made, but in fact it's not credible, it's incredible. Now it's 3:00 A.M. and you're halfway through Layne Norton confusing you on a twenty-five-minute-long YouTube video. You finally peel yourself away from your computer three hours later and none of your questions have been answered, but you're sold.

When it comes to accepting IIFYM as a legitimate diet, think of every other time you had to take a big risk and how you fucking owned it. Like the first time your frail arms put up 135lbs on the bench with no spotter. Remember that moment? Of course you do. Remember why you had to buck up and put up the bar? Because you had no choice. Because it was chest day and you ain't about to bail on those gains. The same goes for IIFYM. You're two breaths away from puking at the sight of chicken and have nowhere else to turn. Take the plunge.

Whoever said, "If it seems too good to be true, it probably is" definitely didn't lift and definitely was not a macro dieter. You can literally have cake and eat cake with IIFYM. This is a no-brainer. Take the plunge. You've come this far so you might as well bust in her because remember, pussy is pussy and a calorie is a calorie.

CHAPTER 32

How to Bulk

"Bulking" is a term used to justify your lack of discipline. In theory, the purpose of bulking is to put on quality muscle mass over the winter in order to shred down over the summer.

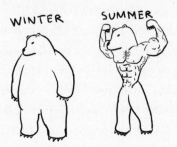

But here at Bro Science, we don't care about theories. We care about facts. And the fact is, bulking is no more than an excuse to be lazy on your diet, improve your bench, and see how much unrestricted low-quality weight you can slop onto your body that'll pass for muscle mass. Sign me up.

Bulking season is always an exciting time of year, at first. You're amped up to eat huge and grow into a meat titan. Then, once your veins and your abs disappear you get cold feet and reconsider your entire life.

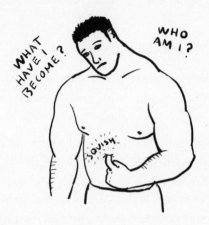

You end up falling into a middle-of-the-road diet where you're not putting on mass or losing fat. By the time summer comes around, you haven't put on enough weight to justify a real cut without wasting away into nothing. When it's all said and done, you just stay the same all year long.

But if this is the year that you tell yourself you're finally going to do a real bulk, then here are two popular bulking methods that I will bro the science right out of.

Clean Bulk

Okay, right off the bat I'm going to tell you that the clean bulk is a myth. Theoretically, a clean bulk consists of strictly consuming clean foods, like grilled chicken, smoked veggies, and air, and, from that, you are expected to gain a bunch of mass. Saying you're going to do a clean bulk is like saying you're going to watch porn but not jerk off. Who do you think you are, the fuckin' pope? Quit lying to yourself, bro. This charade will last three weeks until you realize you physically can't eat six buckets of reheated quinoa and four plates of boiled chicken every day. No one knows if a clean bulk works because no one's ever done it.

If It Fits Your Macros (IIFYM)

You guys know by now that IIFYM is some sort of wizardry of a diet that says you can eat whatever you want as long as it fits your macronutrient requirements. The problem here is, who the fuck actually counts their macros? Who are you, fuckin' Rain Man? "Definitely, definitely lime green Jell-O day. Definitely, definitely 300.4 . . . grams of protein." No way, bro.

Let's take a closer look at IIFYM. I've been strictly adhering to the diet for two months now and am pretty fucking proud of myself. I haven't done this much counting since . . . ever. The other day I had my first slipup. It happens. I'm not mad about it. My boy hit me up during my yearly rest day to go day drinking. Say no more. By 11:00 P.M. we hadn't eaten a damn thing since 9:00 A.M. and needed some fuckin' macros, bro. Boom. IHOP FTW. I'm too drunk to math, so I had to freestyle my macros. Seven pancakes later I figured I'd made up for the lost macros. I fit my macros in. Sometimes it's not a question of if it will fit, but what you are trying to fit it into. Either way, you're gonna find a way to make it fit. You'll always find a way.

In summation, don't let these theories hold you back. If you want to crush seven slices of pizza, wear hoodies, and bench four plates, then fucking do it. That's what bulking is all about. Bulking is freedom. Bulking is America. Bulking is Justice.

CHAPTER 33

How to Cut

Now that you're learned on the art of bulking, it's time to see what's on the other side of the fence. If bulking is that sloppy chick you bang on the DL, super easy, nothing to brag about and you always feel guilty afterward, then cutting is her tight-boxed sister that you ask out every year cuz you think you actually got a shot at getting the keys to the butt house, but really she's just gonna toss you a pity handy and not let you finish. You and I both know you're going back for more, though.

Let's look at the psychology of cutting. At the start of every summer, you tell yourself, "This summer I'm actually going to get shredded. I'm going to have shoulder striations, ab veins, I'm gonna have abs on my fucking dick: #sixcock." But chances are you fall into one of the following categories:

1. Your bulk didn't go so well and now you have a head start on being lean, but you're clinging to any size you managed to gain over the winter.
2. Your bulk went too well and now you're just fat.

Either way, you start to cut because you've convinced yourself for the eighth year in a row that you are going to be the shredded guy this summer. So if you really want to go down this road again, then hop in the car. Spoiler alert: It's a NASCAR and we're driving in circles.

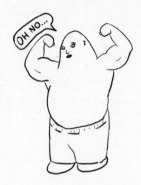

Cutting Carbs

Cutting carbs implies that you are still eating clean, which leaves you with the worst that food has to offer. It's like having access to all the porn in the world, but still jerking off to your imagination. Eating clean is the quickest way to bail on your cut because once you see how flat you look without carbs you'll reconsider every choice you've ever made. There is nothing worse than looking flat. The difference between being flat and being cut or shredded is size and contour. If you're flat, you look and feel like the wind can blow you away at any time. Cutting carbs is like watching the movie *It's a Wonderful Life* in reverse, where the angel shows you what a pussy you look like and makes you want to kill yourself.

IIFYM

You still can't accept that this may actually work. Flexible dieting goes against everything you've based your life on, and now some bro is telling me I can get cut and still eat pizza? What's next, you're gonna tell me that Jesus didn't kill all the dinosaurs? I'm not buying it, guy from the future sent here to fuck with my gains. I don't need to try something new.

Cardio

Ha, ha, nope. Yeah, cardio is a great way to cut, but I'd rather cut my fat with a fucking hacksaw than jump on a treadmill. I bet you're telling yourself, "Sure, cardio is no big deal . . . just twenty minutes post-workout, three times a week, and I'll be shredded." Yeah, it's also no big deal to visit my grandma in the nursing home once a year. Pass. And don't even get me started on fasted cardio. Running while starved, are you kidding me? Here's what's going to happen: You are going to do cardio once, maybe twice, then you are going to convince yourself you actually *shouldn't* do it because it's going to make you even smaller. Especially because you're already looking flat from your accidental gluten-free diet. Cardio and a gluten-free diet . . . congrats, bro. The only thing you cut is your dick off.

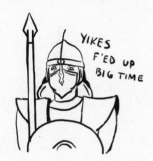

Fat-Burning Supplements

By definition supplements should be supplementing one of the other things on this list. Likely, they are going to be the only tactic you stick with because all you have to do is consume them. So they should no longer be called fat-burning supplements, they should be called fat-burning solutions.

When it comes down to it, there aren't too many ways to cut. It's a slow and unrewarding process because all you want to do is fuel up so you can hit the gym with the same intensity you're used to. So, most likely, this year is still not your year. You thought since you're not the biggest, you'd be the leanest, but you are neither because you are stuck in body purgatory, aka the bro cycle.

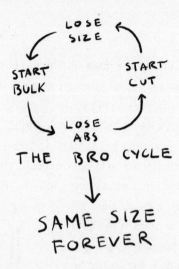

THE BRO CYCLE

SAME SIZE
FOREVER

Every season you are constantly gaining and cutting the same ten pounds. It's like a caterpillar going into a cocoon and coming out as a caterpillar again. Bitches don't wanna fuck no hairy-ass worm. The bitches you prey on can't even see cuts, let's be real, bro. To them, as long as you don't have a gut, you have abs. You might think veins make you look jacked, but girls just think you look like a squeezed ball sack. The only people who give a shit about being 6 percent body fat are dudes, and the only thing that really matters to dudes is who is bigger. If you really wanna win this summer, don't cut the fat, cut the bullshit and cut to the chase. #SummerBulk.

CHAPTER 34

Spring Break

Now we're talking. You and your squad of rabid wolves pooled your cash together over the past year and finally can book that Spring Break Groupon deal. For a meathead, Spring Break is your Mr. Olympia. You have it harder, though. Mr. Olympia is a one-day event. You gotta keep in competition form for an entire week in Mexico while drowning in pussy, alcohol, and the pool. You are ready to showcase the gains you've slaved over in the gym to every sloppy sorority chick you encounter. Fuck it, maybe you'll go after a couple of locals while you're stumbling around at 4:00 A.M. looking for street tacos.

Few events make you lift harder. Spring Break is your Colosseum.

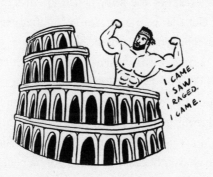

It's the biggest concert in the world, and you're the fucking head-liner. Even better, with all of the alcohol you'll be drinking you'll have a perfect blend of being shredded from dehydration and carbing the fuck up so you can fill up your muscle tanks. This is the perfect marriage of pseudo-leanness and thick-ass bread muscles. Coincidentally this lasts exactly one week. Also, being tan is dope.

BRO FACT: Tans decrease body fat by 11 percent. So get ready for a week of nothing but flexing. Be prepared to have your abs engaged, your shoulders back, and your chest out, ready to pour warm tequila down your throat after a harsh pregame of vodka and pre-workout.

Here's how it goes. Boom. You're fresh off the plane, eight Jack and gingers deep, ready to hit the ground running. Don't get too ahead of yourself, though. You have about two hours of admin to handle before you sip non-plane alcohol. First you get to your room, shower up, and rush over to your friend's room across the hall. He's still in the shower and he's gotta wait for his boys from another school who don't arrive for another three hours. At this point, you're the closest to sober that you'll be this entire trip. Take advantage. Pop your shirt off and do the only bodyweight exercises you know: push-ups and dips between the two hotel beds. Get that pump in. You're looking extra vascular because of all the alcohol you ripped on the plane.

Finally, the entire crew is present. You dap each other up and exchange stories about how hard your frat went at last week's party. It's all smiles because the pool is the plan. All of your priorities and concerns should revolve around what your pump is gonna look like at the pool. If you don't go to the pool with a pump, you might as well give your dick to charity because you ain't gonna be using it. You and the crew head over all juiced up. Turns out you wasted the afternoon in the hotel getting drunk and slapping each other. You show up to the pool. It's 5:00 P.M., a little cloudy, kind of cold, and everyone is shit-faced and headed back to their rooms. Whatever. You take a few seconds to analyze the dudes who are there and how you're bigger than them. Validate yourself and get to drinking. #BroShots.

Next thing you know it's just you and your homie hanging out in the hotel hot tub drinking Mai Tais talking about the destruction that's going to happen tomorrow. Tomorrow's a big day. It's the booze cruise. You have your freshest ocean gear full of American flags and Greek lettering already laid out. Plus, your entire crew got matching sunglasses from your boy who started a sunglasses company in San Diego. So sick.

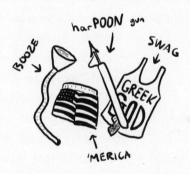

You wake up so hungover. Feels like you've been smacked in the head with a frying pan all night. You have drunk zero water and your mouth feels like you ate a bag of wood chips. You open your eyes to see your boy passed out facedown on the floor and know this is going to be the trip legends are made of. First things first: Throw on your gear and hit the hotel bar before the bus leaves for the booze cruise. You got the wristband, so you're going to clean up the bar. Nothing like 9:00 A.M. daiquiris and some weird Mexican granola bars you don't remember buying.

Once you hit the boat you start fading. It hits you that you're already shithoused, extremely tired, jet-lagged, scarily dehydrated, and about to embark on three hours of trying to grind on chicks to EDM while on a boat. This is a blessing in disguise. Two minutes in and you're leaning over the edge of the boat violently yakking into the ocean. Four more sessions and you feel cleansed. Time to show everyone what you're about. Funnel a beer and hit the dance floor despite everyone telling you that you look like death.

You blink a couple times and the cruise is over. You have no idea what the past two hours consisted of, but once you step foot on dry land you are immediately in need of a survival kit. Make the bus driver stop at the next convenience store, where you grab a tall can of Red Bull and an entire loaf of whole wheat bread. No water. You go straight to your room, sit on the edge of the bed, and eat the entire loaf while you wait for your bros to shower. No time for naps. Cabs leave for the club in two hours.

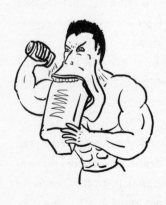

Whoa, you need some play money. Your debit card has dollars on it, but this ATM only gives out pesos. #FreeMoney #BeatingTheSystem #PyramidScheme. You already spent all your pesos on duty-free novelty shot glasses from the airport, which you broke last night. Now you're in the cab line alone. Your boys ditched you and got their own cab, now you gotta jump in with three random uggos who spend the entire ride talking about how they originally majored in Psych at UDel but switched to Marketing and can't wait to kill it at this summer's internship.

Go time. You arrive at the club. It's an empty fucking warehouse, but you know it's about to look like last year's Hardwell Coachella tent. As always, you and the boys came correct. You threw in $200 extra each for bottle service at a private table overlooking the dance floor.

This is going to be your first bottle service experience and you're envisioning a rap video full of champagne and strippers. Turns out instead of champagne you get the cheapest vodka possible. Straight poison. You think you aren't even getting drunk from chugging the bottle, then all of a sudden it hits. Wasted. You're tongue-deep in one of the now shoeless uggos you took the cab over with because, coincidentally, she's the only chick you've spoken to this entire trip.

You realize your shirt has been on the whole time. What the hell is wrong with you? You pound your chest and rip off your Express button-down. Your boys are cheering you on. You're certain this act solidifies a handy from this chick. You step away to craft her another cocktail of ice, vodka, and a splash of water. The moment you look up she's nowhere to be found. Spring Break took her. Another one bites the dust.

Your entire squad is blacked out beyond belief for the second time in one day. How is this possible? Somehow you make it back to your room and pass out with your contacts in. You don't even wear contacts. You wake up in the morning with porn on your iPhone. There's only wifi in the lobby, so looks like you had to 3G that nut. This is gonna cost you, like, $600. You don't even know if you nutted. Oh . . . yeah . . . you did. You definitely nutted. Flood in the basement.

Now that you're up, there's no chance of going back to sleep. There's already heavy Weezy blaring from neighboring rooms and you're catching some 9:00 A.M. FOMO. You think about showering, but remember there's a pool. Good enough. Hit the buffet beforehand, shovel down some cold scrambled eggs and a couple breakfast brews.

BRO TIP: Start drinking before your body realizes it's hungover. Beat it to the punch with punch, beer punch, aka beer and orange juice.

This is your first full day at the pool, so you're gonna storm over there like it's D-Day at Normandy. Before anything even happens, you're four tequila shots deep. Spring Break shots are like blinking: You don't try to do it but it's always happening. Now you've found yourself in a circle of people. You know none of them, but you're all best friends for life, you swear. You "Cheers" to anything and everything, sometimes twice. You're all screaming unbelievable requests at the bartender who can't speak English and has to feed his family off the tips you're giving him. Every time you step away from the circle, you return with a round of drinks for the *familia*. You feel like you're part of the *Fast and Furious* crew.

This process repeats itself for seven more days. You lose track of time and feel like you're a citizen of Mexico. This feels like home. You even got a haircut from the local barber. Don't get too comfortable. A couple of blinks later, you wake up hungover and realize your plane leaves in an hour. You catch a glimpse of yourself in the mirror and realize there is no time for good-byes. Sure, you're the most shredded you've ever been, but you're also a twig.

All those months of cutting, and bulking and cutting and bulking over and over . . .

You wonder, Was this all worth it? Terrible question: You know it was. Your Spring Break was so legendary your fans can smell the tequila through your social media. Take a second to appreciate this moment and how far you've come. Happy? Good. Because it's time to get back into the fucking gym, you skinny bitch. You don't have much time, summer is only a few weeks away.

STAGE 5

Gym Rat

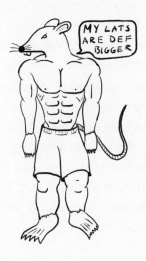

Congratulations are in order: You have officially taken shape. Take a minute to think about what you once were and where you are now. We all started as primordial ooze, but some of us kept evolving, like you.

At this point, dudes are actually coming up to you in the gym and asking how you got your triceps to look like that. When you go home for Thanksgiving break, you are *the* hometown hero. Sometimes you're even keeping a button-down on long enough to unveil those cannons after a single beer, because you barely drink anymore. Empty calories. You will stop in the middle of a crowded street to catch a glimpse of your reflection in a store window. Better yet, if the lighting is right, your shirt is coming off and it's a one-man photo shoot. You no longer practice competition poses in your bathroom, but out in the open, in front of your roommates, who now fucking hate you, but you can't tell because you can't see them. They can definitely see you. Because you are the human form of glory.

At this point you have achieved women, yet you spend all your time in the gym surrounded by other dudes just like you. Your competitive instincts kick in and you develop the urge to be the biggest dude wherever you go. You are constantly sizing up other dudes and the details of their body. You compare yourself to every guy and you are constantly unhappy with yourself and all that you've achieved to this point. I'm so proud. You are a certified meathead. You have eaten, lived, and breathed Bro Science and are now brofessor to many brotégés whose first names you don't know.

You are moving at a rapid pace through the evolution of the lifting man. Read on to find out how to maximize your gain potential. Learn simple mental exercises like how to make sure that your mind doesn't even think about taking a rest day and how to get a pump while you're at home doing everyday activities. Go forth, swoldier.

CHAPTER 35

New Gym Checklist

Okay, you just joined a new gym and are about to hit your first workout. Don't expect to just walk in and jump into your workout like it's your old gym. You're the new kid at school and if you don't play your cards right, before you know it you'll be the kid that's sexually aroused by dragons playing four square by himself at recess. You really wanna be the kid that never changes for gym class? Didn't think so. Your first workout is all about posturing. You wanna try really fucking hard to look cool without looking like you're trying really fucking hard to look cool. Follow this new gym checklist to make sure you'll be sitting with the cool kids.

Make sure your gym doesn't say Planet Fitness. Planet Fitness prides itself on not pushing its patrons to get fucking huge. That's not a place you want to be in.

Rock your best gym outfit. Make sure it's freshly laid out for you the night before. I'm talkin' the best gear no one's even seen yet. You gotta drop a couple benjamins at the Nike store? No problem, put it on the credit card. You'll pay off your debt in swag.

Pre-workout. Take the maximum dosage. This is like popping Viagra before your prom. You can get the job done without it but you wanna stack the odds and swing the bone hammer. It's not a question of how much should you take, it's a question of how much can you take.

Score a primo parking spot. This is your grand entrance. You want everyone to see you drive up and take the stage before you get inside and realize you have no idea where the fuck you are.

Pull the "I don't know what the fuck I'm doing" bicep pump. This accomplishes two things: 1. You can scope out the gym without standing around looking like a noob and 2. You a grab a nectar bicep pump before you move about the gym and are seen and immediately judged. Judged by how huge your arm cannons are.

Have a plan. Don't ever look lost. If the piece of equipment you plan to use next gets taken don't panic, and most of all, do not stand around with your thumb up your ass. This is the equivalent of standing in the middle of the lunchroom holding your tray. You might as well wear a sign that says "I still have lice." Jump on the nearest piece of equipment and start doing curls.

Find the biggest dude.

Make sure that dude is you. They say if you are the most successful person in the room, then find a new room. If you are the biggest dude in the room, then make that room your gym.

Maintain hard face: The key to looking cool is looking completely unapproachable. Weird thing is, when someone starts talking to you your voice becomes softer than a lamb's orgasm.

Go heavy. Even though their eyes aren't on you and they don't even know you're there, trust me, everyone's looking at you. You're under the microscope. Give 'em something big to look at.

See if it's cool to take your shirt off. And by "see" I mean take it off wherever there are the most mirrors and put up some weight.

Find the best lighting. There's one spot in every gym that has lighting like a real-life Instagram filter. Find this spot. Do all your lifts here.

Engage selfie stealth mode on your phone. Sound off, flash off. If you're lifting you're going to be taking selfies, this is a law of nature like Fibonacci and shit. But don't get busted snapping selfies if you're the new guy.

Do some random show-off workouts that have nothing to do with your current workout. Whatever your strongest exercise is, just fucking do it. Anything to show off. If you're working back but you can bang out hundos on shoulder press, grab a couple sets. If you can bang out muscle ups but know damn well they have nothing to do with any of your workouts, what are you waiting for?

Wrap up with some cardio. This will be the first and last time you do cardio in this gym. Do it for the ladies. Show them you're well rounded.

⫘—⫘

Follow my steps and that gym will be yours by the end of your session. Every chick in the gym is going to chase after you asking for your autograph as you walk to your car. Give them a smile and tell them you'll be back tomorrow, twice.

CHAPTER 36

How to Get Hyped for a Lift

Listen, even Zeus had days when the last thing he fucking wanted to do was go to the gym. You're only human, bro. We've all been in that place when you're on a thirty-six-day gym streak, but nothing sounds better than eating some bar nachos, pouring pitchers of Bud Light down your throat, and talking to chicks about how sick your tailgates are. You can't help it; we all have needs. Lifting heavy-ass weight and being a fucking truck house is hard.

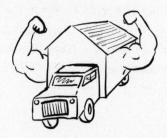

Sometimes when pure might, animal strength, four rounded scoops of Gnar Pump, and crippling inadequacy issues aren't enough to complete a lift, you need to find ways to gain that mental edge and mind fuck your brain pussy into beast mode.

When it comes to lifting, your brain is your best worst friend.

Your brain is that one bro you have that's always pushing you to do shit you shouldn't, like, "Yo, you can def clear that pong table longways" when he knows your body is physically not the one for the job. Without your brain, you're a vegetable, and vegetables are for runners and that annoying vegan chick spamming your Instagram feed: #EatWithIntention. Use your brain to constantly remind your body that it isn't good enough and needs to be in the gym when you have one of those days where all you wanna do is crush the new Destiny on Xbox for twelve hours straight. Don't go running off using your brain muscles for books and word sandwiches and shit. Use it to lift heavy things. Here are some methods to hype yourself up and get that mental pump.

Pre-Gym Pump Porn

Cue up YouTube and watch some dude that you admire a little bit too much physically and look up to a little bit too much emotionally. His spiritual rants and/or threats to your life will make you think you can get to his level, and this will keep you motivated just long enough to blast out a few hard lifts, roughly equal to the time it takes reality to set in.

Pre-Workout

When nature just isn't enough, the mystery chemicals and shiny words on every pre-workout canister will inject strength directly into your body via triple blue explosion berry.

The Walk Around

The hardest part is over: You've actually made it to the gym. Now circle your weight like a shark circling its prey. Mutter crazy shit, bang your fists together, and let the weights know about their impending doom. It's not a rest for you, it's a rest for your weights.

Go to Smackdonald's

Pain is an excellent motivator. Remember, you're on the path to becoming a Freak Beast. Soon you will start looking more animal than man, and it's time to start behaving like one. You want to walk into the zoo and be led straight to your cage, with the other gorillas. So get angry. Smack yourself. Wake your muscles up the old-fashioned way, by smacking yourself—but not by doing actual smack. Come on, bro. If you don't want to abuse yourself, get your best bro to start smacking your chest and your arms. There is zero doubt that this will piss you off and get the blood flowing through your veins like fresh lava. You're going to want to throw up so much weight the entire gym will shut down. Violence is the answer.

The Muscle Monk

Huddle over your weights like you're praying for forgiveness for these sins you're about to commit.

See ya in fuckin' church. Head down and stare at yourself in the mirror under your eyebrows. You look like Scorpion from Mortal Kombat. Mentally tell yourself how badass you are.

The Coach

When it's not enough to just think it and do it, verbally tell your body what to do. Let small incomplete phrases slip out through your breathing. Don't worry about getting loud with it; you're going to bang around so much weight in a few minutes that no one will be the wiser.

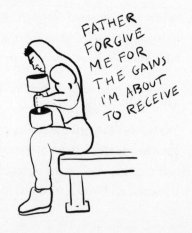

FATHER FORGIVE ME FOR THE GAINS I'M ABOUT TO RECEIVE

The One-Upper

You're a highly competitive beast whose entire existence revolves around one-upping. Get that gym motivation by letting your bro go first, then grabbing whatever weight is the next heaviest for your set. Put it up and put him down. Your ego is doing the legwork here, and by legwork, I mean chest work.

The Beat Dropper

Crush your workout to the private rave you have going on in your head. Crank the volume up full blast for your first few sets to set the workout in motion. This beat drop is your moment. Everyone will be saying, "Yo bro, that was sick how you banged out that lift right when the beat dropped! You're a real cool guy and also much bigger than me as well. You should compete." Aren't you glad you got up off the couch?

The Show-Off

This is self-explanatory: You put on the show and they get off. Nothing gets you hyped like blasting out 65lb incline dumbbell press next to a chick just passing by who doesn't even notice you on her way to the exit to blow her boyfriend who lifts more than you. #PussyWizard.

The Yell

The weights have been bad, they need to be spanked . . . with your mouth. Yell at them. Scare the weights . . . and the people around you. The adrenaline you'll build up from being a huge spectacle will carry you through the lift, no problem.

Stretch Armstrong

Nothing prepares you for a lift like violent stretches that lead to sick shoulder impingement. People are going to be watching you stretch so aggressively that they'll be scared about what's going to happen afterward, but they're going to watch to be a part of the spectacle. Build up the anticipation of your onlookers with your intense stretches and foam rolling. By the time you set up for your first rep your fans will be cheering from the sidelines.

The Intra-Workout Supp Guy

You look like a complete tool, but you are getting a ton of placebo energy from that ambiguous pink liquid stinking up the entire gym with each sip. Keep it up and be sure to renew your gold card at GNC. Chump.

The Sneak Attack

Remember, you have a brain, the weights don't. Lift the weights before gravity has a chance to make them heavy. The element of surprise comes before Iron on the periodic table.

The Asshole Shadow Boxer

Revenge is the greatest motivator. Before you grab any iron, stand in front of the dumbbell rack and fight back the ghosts of the people who are stronger than you. Stare at yourself in the mirror, so everyone can see that the champ is in the building. Keep punching, Muhammad Small-i.

The Captive Spotter

Grab a random dude that you want to prove yourself to and make him spot you. Ha, joke's on him. He can't help but spot you with his eyes.

You got this dude 'mirin'. His validation is like that extra scoop of pre-workout mid-set.

⊪—⊪

Now that you know the secrets to gym motivation, you have no reason to ever take a rest day. So the next time your side chick hits you with the "You home?" smash text and you're on your couch doing nothing but thinking about how you should be at the gym, you best hit her back with, "Naw, heading to the gym."

CHAPTER 37

Why Rest Days Are Bullshit

If you're like me, the only way to force yourself to rest is to physically handcuff yourself to your couch, with real police handcuffs that you don't have the key to. #ArrestDay. Now, before I attempt muscle suicide by staying in here all day, let me tell you why rest days are bullshit.

First of all, what is a rest day? It's a day taken off from lifting to allow your body to, allegedly, but definitely not, recover and build muscle. It's pretty much a day spent in a coma. "Rest" means three things:

1. The act of stagnant rotting.
2. The shit nobody wants. It's like, "Hey, bro, you want the rest of this shit?" No I don't want the rest.
3. Idle hands are the devil's playthings, which means if you rest, the devil is gonna use your hands to jerk himself off. Is that what you want?

Before you answer that, let's think about who rests: idiot babies, saggy geezers, and the mentally unstable. Ipso facto, rest is for the weak. When you work out, you get stronger, so what the hell are you resting from? I don't have weekdays on my calendar, only strongdays.

BRO MATH: 7 strong days in a strong, 4 strongs a month, 52 strongs a year.

DOMCEMBER

M	T	W	T	F	S	S
1 STRONG	2 STRONG	3 STRONG	4 STRONG	5 STRONG	6 STRONG	7 STRONG
8 STRONG	9 STRONG	10 STRONG	11 STRONG	12 STRONG	13 STRONG	14 STRONG
15 STRONG	16 STRONG	17 STRONG	18 STRONG	19 STRONG	20 STRONG	21 STRONG
22 STRONG	23 STRONG	24 STRONG	25 STRONG	26 STRONG	27 STRONG	28 STRONG
29 STRONG	30 STRONG	31 STRONG				

If you follow this method, before you know it, you'll literally have no more weekdays in your life, too.

People who say rest days are important are straight-up ignorant. They are dark age simpletons who claim you build muscle when you rest. Okay, smart guy, if this is true . . . then what about sloths? Checkmate. Three-pointer for the win, and it was a dunk.

Resting does not mean that you have to take an entire day of rest. It just means that when you are not in the gym, you should *always* be resting. Have a job interview at your dad's accounting firm? Hand in your two weeks' notice during the interview, cuz the only thing you're counting from now on is how many hours of rest to squeeze in before you hit the gym. Found true love? Guess again, Jennifer Aniston, because you're married to the game. Got other hobbies or interests? We both know you don't. You're a Gym Rat, not a gym dolphin. You don't have any other tricks up your sleeve, cuz you don't wear sleeves. You only got one thing on your mind: Where's the fuckin' cheese? That shredded cheddar. That pepper jacked #ARMesan.

Some people will tell you you're overtraining. These haters don't want to see people do better than them.

> **BRO FACT:** Every time you get bigger, someone else gets smaller. No one's going to help you make them smaller; they are going to tell you to rest. Overtraining is like global warming—the only people that bitch about it are the ones who can't stand the heat. Fact of the matter is, I'd rather overtrain than under gain.

The worst part about a rest day is being alone with yourself without a pump. You love yourself if and only if you have a pump. It's those days when you're alone with your deflated self that you realize a pump is all you have going for yourself. It's like being in public without your phone. What are you going to do now? Be forced to talk to people? No way, bro.

You wanna take a rest day? Let me tell you how to take a proper rest day:

Do only seated exercises.

Train the *rest* of the muscles you always forget to hit, like abs, calves, forearms—anything but legs. That's when you take a rest day.

Follow my workout split:

Monday: chest

Tuesday: arms

Wednesday: arms

Thursday: chest

Friday: arms

Saturday: chest and arms

Sunday: rest and arms

You are on the way to becoming one of the greats. One of the humans that only comes around once in a lifetime. You are the living example of what hard work, for, like, two hours a day, looks like. You think Steve Jobs or Mother Teresa could put up the weight you do? No shot. It's all on you. You actually have weight on your shoulders because it's shoulder day. The only thing you have in common with the best of the best is that you don't fucking rest. You have the unmatched determination to sacrifice normal human existence, fortune, and fame to wake up at 11:00 A.M. every day, wear sweatpants all day, and work out around 3:00 P.M. Every. Single. Day. And it shows, bro. Because you are looking huge.

Now that you know how to properly rest when you're not ripping up the Boneyard, read on to get learned on the best ways to grab a pump from home.

CHAPTER 38

Extreme Pump Secrets—Home Edition

You just got back from the gym, what are you gonna do? Play video games? No. You're going to superset your gym sesh with an at-home workout. Just because you leave the gym doesn't mean you're no longer a meathead. A true meathead brings his work home with him.

Think of yourself as a single father with six kids: Biceps, Triceps, Chest, Back, Shoulders, and Abs. Oh, Legs, too. Always forget about them. Joint custody: I only see them every other weekend, if that.

Caring for these muscle children is a full-time job. My muscles are my number-one concern. Once I leave the gym I'm already thinking about my next pump. Eighty percent of my day is spent worrying that I'm looking flat, the other 15 percent is spent learning percentages. A true Bro Scientist is all about sneaking in those secret pumps. Here are a few ways to snag those secret pumps at home or at, as I like to call it, my gym away from gym.

Biceps

Mankind's sole purpose is to discover ways of keeping your bicep pump. There have been deep-sea explorations devoted to searching for ancient bicep pump secrets below the earth's surface, yet there's one hiding right in your laundry basket. Let's say you're heading out to do some laundry. Just grab that hamper and sneak in some curls. Maybe there'll be some honeys in the laundry room. #CurlsForTheGirls

Triceps

Triceps are the biceps of the back of your arms. If you're getting a bicep pump, rest assured you're gonna want a tricep pump. It's like taking protein. You always want two scoops, but you can't do two scoops with just one scoop. Here's a great tip for that tricep pump: Swiffer your floors real hard. If you've ever Swiffered before, you know how hard you gotta push down to get those floors clean. Fifteen minutes of Swiffering and your triceps are gonna make your biceps jealous.

Back

Science has yet to confirm if it's possible to achieve a back pump, but what does science know anyway? You want a secret back pump? Try on a lot of shirts. Any type of shirt will do. The up-and-down motion of putting a T-shirt on over and over will get your lats right. Trying to fit into that new button-down that's two sizes too small involves the pulling motion needed to get that turtle shell. All that's left is calling your boy into the room to ask him to snap some pics of your back pump because you just proved science wrong.

Traps and Forearms

Traps and forearms are body ornaments, straight-up decoration muscles. Nothing says Swolbroham Lincoln like having a thick neck and pumped forearms. You want a trap and forearm pump? Carry all your groceries in at once. Show everyone in your building how strong you are. You see an old woman or a weaker man pushing a shopping cart to the car? Get your ass over there, take the bags out of the cart, and do a sick farmer's carry all the way to the car. You're going to pump your traps, improve your posture, and win the hearts of all the chicks who wished their boyfriends were more like you.

Shoulders

When you have a good shoulder pump you feel like nothing's wide enough for you, which it isn't. It's like, fuck it, you might just rock a cutoff to the club and sleep in an airplane hangar. For that nasty shoulder pump, superset five minutes of shampooing with three minutes of conditioner. Do this for four sets and you won't be able to fit out of the shower.

Chest

Hugs. No out-of-gym movement engages all parts of your chest like a good old-fashioned hug. Remember, this is for the pump and nothing else. Find the nearest human and wrap your arms around them like you're trying to cut off all the circulation to their brain. Your chest is going to pop out of your shirt and the person you hugged will be thankful to have such a good muscle friend.

Legs

You want a leg pump, for whatever reason? This is a no-brainer: Take the stairs. Internet memes say that friends don't let friends skip leg day. I'm not sure where you found your friends, but you should probably find some new ones or just do what I do and not have any. Looks like I'm taking the elevator. #PentHoused #69thFloor.

Bosu Ball

Wanna tighten up those abs before you hit the club? Kill two birds with one stone. Masturbate on an exercise ball. *Flex nut!*

Follow my pump secrets and you'll have people 'mirin' 24/7. My findings have been tested by yours truly for the same amount of time it takes to become a doctor. So consider me Dr. Mazzetti, MD (Most Diesel). If any of you Gym Rats out there have any pump secrets of your own, be sure to mail them to me via Twitter @BroScienceLife.

CHAPTER 39

How to Fix Injuries and Imbalances

At this stage, you're addicted to the gym and you never want to rest, but you're starting to discover problems that arose from years of lifting without proper form. Fuck it. There's no going back now, you gotta be alpha all the time. The natural progression.

A lot of brotégés have been hitting me up on social media, asking me if injuries are real, and their questions got me thinking. For the first seven years of my lifting career, the only injuries I had were the ones I made up to get out of leg day. So no, I didn't believe that injuries were real. But now that I'm a little older and my joints grind harder than the bottle thots in the club . . . well, I still don't believe injuries are real. Anything or anyone that gets in the way of my gym time has no time in my reality. That popping sound? That's not an injury, that's just my joints clapping for me. Injuries are your muscles pushing bones out of the way to make space for themselves.

Lemme bring you back to the beginning. You started training through Bro Science. Your brofessor just grabbed you from the pound and threw you into the ring with the big dogs. He's been lifting since his dad forced him to join Pee Wee football and day one you jumped right into his workout, mainly because he needed a spot. But you never built a foundation. You saw a plot of land and you dropped a house on it like you were playing Monopoly. Ten years later you step back and look at the house you built and realize . . . this shit is crooked as hell. You should have spent more time building the foundation. Now you're looking like a juiced-up Quasimodo. But the past is the past. You are now faced with two choices: Tear the house down and build that foundation right, or live larger and make the house bigger.

I would actually rather build an entire house from scratch than try to rebuild my body. Nothing is worse than fixing your body's foundation, because it involves stretching. Everyone talks about how good stretching is, but have you ever seen a ripped muscle god do it? No way, bro. Stretching is like taking a cycle off of pre-workout. You know you should've cycled off sixteen months ago, but you're going to do it next week instead, or the week after. Like, it's cool to be flexible if you're a chick cuz you can turn into a sex transformer in bed. But if you're a dude, what are you gonna do? Throw your leg behind your head while you're stickin' her with that sick mish? No chick wants to see what horrors are hiding behind your nutsack. It's like fuckin' Mordor down there, man.

Lemme guess, now you're gonna ask me whether you should start foam rolling. Maybe you complained about the nagging back pain you've had, and you were overheard by some gym shaman; the fucking spiritual healer of the gym. (Not to be confused with Top Ramen, the noodles of the kitchen.) Now, Rafiki over here tells you to try foam rolling. Who the fuck do you think you're talking to, bro? Foam rolling is bullshit. I've been rolling since house music was called techno. Save your lectures for that group of dudes in the Total Body Sculpt class at 6:30 P.M.

If you accept that you have a problem and decide you want to try to fix your injuries and imbalances then you're looking at tacking another thirty minutes of not lifting into your workout, which could be spent hitting calves, which I didn't do in the first place because I used that extra thirty minutes for more sets of bench. But now I'm definitely not doing calves. Now I'll never have big calves. So I might as well keep benching.

So yeah, my house may be crooked, but this is America and you're damn right I'm going to keep making my house bigger and bigger until all the neighbors move the fuck out of my neighborhood. I'd rather be the Leaning Tower of Pisa than the perfectly straight bitch house of nobody gives a fuck.

CHAPTER 40

How to Be Alpha All the Time

You are a lion, and the gym is your kingdom. So how are you supposed to let people know about your muscles when they can't see your pump or don't know how much you can lift? Not even Einstein can answer that. But I can. The golden rule of being a forever alpha is to make sure you are flexing at all times. There are tons of opportunities to flex throughout the day when you're not in the gym. The goal is to be flexing so often that your body won't ever return to its unflexed state. It's like facing a bottle of Viagra that lasts forever.

When Applying Deodorant

Pop that shirt off, stare grimly into the mirror, and watch your lats pop as you apply. Have a bro snap a pic for maximum exposure.

Brushing Your Teeth

Another bathroom gem. Push the brush hard into your gums; if you draw blood that means you're doing it right. If you snap your toothbrush in half that means you're definitely getting laid tonight.

Leaning on Things

When you lean on absolutely everything possible, you are telling the world how exhausted you are from crushing the gym all week. Best of all, you don't need to tell them with words. They are witnessing the greatness happen right in front of them. If you knock over a bookshelf or two, good.

Reading a Book

Don't actually read the book, just hold it really tight so your forearms bulge out. Every time you turn a page, rip it out, because you are too strong to hold paper.

Taking a Nap

You grow in your sleep, so make sure you look alpha as fuck when it's lights-out. Lay on your back and engage full body flex. You'll eventually pass out from sheer exhaustion.

When Someone Pulls Up Next to You in a Car, Hit 'Em with the Three Pointer

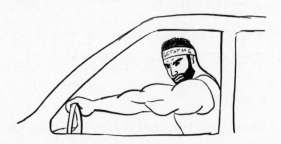

The three pointer is when you grip the steering wheel with your left arm so your forearm is exposed. Your entire arm will be engaged, and your tricep so big the sun will get scared. Fuck it, your traps are going to be flexed out and your neck will look like some grated cheddar.

When You Shake Someone's Hand, Look Directly at Your Own Arm

You stopped caring about establishing eye contact the moment you started lifting. We all know, with arms like yours, where everyone's eyes go anyway. You're like the chick in high school who came back after summer break with titty implants.

Use a Cocktail Shaker Even If You Don't Know How to Make a Cocktail

It's a shake weight for booze.

If You Drop Something, Deadlift It Back Up

This doesn't have to be an accident either. Whoops, you just happened to drop a couple of garbage bags full of filled-up water bottles in front of that chick down the hallway . . . how convenient.

Don't Open Doors, Row Doors

This one has been right in front of you your entire life. You will never open the door the same way again, and for good reason. Who cares if your crew is already inside the club? Not you. You're getting four sets of rows in.

Get Out of a Pool as Many Times as Possible

Doesn't get much better than this. An actual reason to pop your shirt off, plus water-resistance training. Engage your arms, tighten your core, poke that chest out, and push out of the pool like the entire world is watching.

Always Offer to Help Your Bro Move, Even If He's Not Moving

If you're a normal person, moving furniture sucks. If you're a superhuman, moving furniture is pure opportunity. Whenever your bro offers to lend a hand with that huge couch you voluntarily started moving, just toss him your phone and tell him to Snapchat that shit. Push it straight to your story.

One-Up Everyone on Literally Anything

Just as you have a bunch of opportunities to physically flex during the day, you also have plenty of chances to flex your ability to do better at everything than everyone else. Learn to one-up any chance you get. Life is one big PR for everyone to witness. For instance, when you're walking up stairs, don't just skip one stair, skip two stairs. You'll feel a good stretch in your hamstrings and it'll be fun winning against everyone else at the mall. Trust me, they'll be talking about you for years.

Always Remind People of Your Lifestyle and How Big You Are, in Case Their Eyes Forgot

Always carry your gym bag. A workout is always imminent in your world. If you're still in school, throw your Jansport in the trash and punch the shit out of your locker until it's unusable. Throw every single textbook into your oversized duffel to maximize pump value. Now you're walking around with, like, 100lbs all day, every day.

Make every shirt you have into a cutoff. Even a vest. At this stage you are doing the world a service by letting them witness your gains.

Make it seem like it's harder for you to fit through things than it actually is. You may be able to back your car out of your mom's garage no problem, but there's no way in hell you can walk through it.

Take up more space then you need. Because you need it. If you're in the locker room, make it really difficult for other dudes to come within five feet of you. It's not weird, it's necessary.

Don't forget to let everyone know how hard-core your diet is by making your protein shake in public whenever possible. Bonus points for interrupting conversations while doing it.

Bring a gallon jug wherever you go, but always keep it only one-eighth full. Filling it with water is always a start, but bring it home with some BCAAs to keep onlookers on their toes.

Eat your reheated Tupperware meals in front of other people. "Sorry bro, gotta eat, can't wait . . . anabolic window. Keep talking, even though I can't even taste this. You want some? Nah, you won't like it. Don't have enough anyways."

⫘—⫘

Just like my at-home pump workouts, being alpha all of the time isn't very difficult. Opportunity is all around you if you're willing to take it. Sure, you may lose some friends here and there, but you will gain gains, and those are your friends for life.

CHAPTER 41

Most Alpha Chest Exercises

So you're heading to the gym to beat your chest like King Kong with angina, but you have no idea what exercises you're going to do. Let's be real for a sec, who the fuck creates lifting routines anymore? Give it a rest, Jim Stoppani. You're a Gym Rat now. You discovered the Bodybuilding.com workout database in the Tadpole stage.

If you're a true bro, your idea of a creating a workout routine involves walking straight into the gym and improvising a jam sesh. Just like your idea of romance is adding your latest Tinder match on Snapchat and warming up the conversation with a fresh shirtless selfie. #YouGetTheFull10SecondsBaby. You're a man; you ain't got time to plan shit. The only plan you got is Plan B.

So when it comes to freestyling a workout you're gonna choose exercises based on two factors: effectiveness and alpha-ness. Effective exercises are exercises that work that you should be doing, like front raises. Alpha exercises are exercises that get you huge that you always feel like doing, like bench. Here are the best chest exercises for looking alpha.

Incline Dumbbell Press

Incline dumbbell is supposed to be harder than flat bench dumbbell because of the angle you're pushing from, but you're a freak of nature, and for some inconceivable reason, you are actually stronger on incline. So you always choose incline because you are stronger on incline, and you're stronger on incline because you never do flat . . . because you always do incline . . . because you're stronger on incline. See what I'm saying? And here's where it gets super alpha . . . people don't know that you are stronger on incline, so when they see you blasting out 80s on incline they're thinking, this guy's gotta do 100s on flat. And just like that, you're benching 100s with 80lb dumbbells. #LifeHack.

Cable Flies

Cable flies are all show, ipso facto, very alpha. Let me break it down.

You are literally the center of attention. You are claiming both sides of one of the most popular and versatile pieces of equipment in the gym. You can do a ton of different exercises with the cables, but you are only ever doing one.

When you prepare to do cable flies you look like you're celebrating a win onstage. You look like Jesus on the cross, but more swole. To execute the movement correctly, pull the cables in like you're grabbing a pair of thots for a brainstorm, and bring 'em into the Thunderdome. If you look closely, you'll notice everyone in the gym is 'mirin'. You should start chargin' them for this show.

Weighted Dips

It doesn't get much more alpha than weighted dips: You're adding weight to your body by a chain hanging from your dick to do an exercise that people can't do with the weight hanging from their bones.

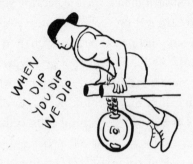

Throw your chain on, ascend the ladder, and dip your 90-pound nutsack into earth's mouth. Django Chained.

And Lastly, the Most Alpha of All Exercises, Bench

Having to explain why bench is alpha is like having to explain why masturbating feels good. A) You're creepy for asking and B) If you have to ask, then you've never done it. There's a reason why "How much can you bench?" has just edged out "What's your name?" for most popular question in the world. It's because no one gives a shit what your name is unless it starts with 315, which makes it first in the *alpha*bet.

CHAPTER 42

Most Alpha Back Exercises

Back might not be the most exciting body part to lift. In fact, Bro Scientists have stated that back is the legs of the upper body, meaning I'll usually skip it for a cooler body part like arms or chest . . . or chest and arms. But what back lacks in being chest, it makes up for in pure strength and residual bicep pump. There's not much to think about, just grab something and pull it; basically, back is the hand job of workouts. So if you want to nut all over back's tits, then do these alpha back exercises and let the gym know the boss is here for business.

Pull-ups

Pull-ups are one of the toughest exercises for regular people to do. But since you're a seasoned lifter at a solid 165lbs, 100lbs of which is waist up, you can bang out pull-ups like nothing is holding you down, like your legs. When you grab the pull-up bar people stop what they are doing and wait to critique your form; they want to see you fail. So when you bang out more than 10 pull-ups with good form, you'll be stuntin' on all those plebeians. If you really want to flex on these commoners, crush some weighted pull-ups. Doing weighted pull-ups is like saying "I am too strong for my own body."

Lat Pulldown

Racking the lat pulldown is like pulling Excalibur from that rock or like lifting Thor's hammer. The closer you can get to the bottom of the stack, the more alpha you become. Make sure to constantly check the dude on the lat pulldown next to you to see where his pin is. You won't be able to make out the numbers, but just make sure your pin is deeper. Wait for him to finish his set then pull out your toaster and serve him up alpha sandwich.

Dumbbell Row

It's easy to hate the dude working out off the dumbbell rack, unless that guy is you, which it is, and you're doing DB rows. Quick nature lesson: What do animals in the wild do when they want to be the alpha male? They beat the shit out of the current alpha, then land his chick while the herd watches. This is how you do a dumbbell row. Stand in front of some dude's mirror space, mount the rack, and butt fuck the dumbbell he was using for bench. Stare at yourself in the mirror as your new pack watches behind you and bows down to their king.

Cable Row

One of the sickest exercises to see yourself doing. Except to see yourself doing it you have to look at a mirror to the side of you. I will gladly jeopardize my neck health to watch this one-man pump orgy go down.

Deadlifts

Some people say deadlifts are for back day, some people say they're for leg day, I say they are for another day. Don't feel like deadlifting today. Pass.

Barbell Row

This is probably the heaviest back exercise you do. Load on the plates and forget about form. Just let it rip. It's not like you are bending over in a vulnerable position dangling weight from your torso and yanking it toward your spine while supporting yourself with just your lower back, ya know, since your hamstrings are closer to string cheese than a normal person's hamstrings. Start the lift with a deadlift so people think you're just going to deadlift that weight. Psych! You're rowing that shit. Bring Ashton Kutcher in here, cuz all you bitches just got Punk'd. If the weight is too heavy to actually bend over, don't lower the weight, just lean forward slightly and do a bent arm shrug. The key here is short T. rex–like movements.

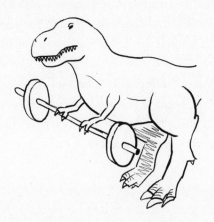

Row row row your back, violently in the gym, bro.

Hit the exercises above and you're going to feel results. You're going to feel huge when you leave the gym and you won't know why, because you can't see your back, but that doesn't mean that chick who's standing behind you in line at Chipotle ain't staring a hole through your lats. Win.

CHAPTER 43

Least Alpha Exercises

Almost all exercises serve a purpose, but that doesn't mean you should be doing them. It's like an adult riding a bicycle with a helmet on. Who are you? Robin Arryn from *Game of Thrones*? You still get breast fed, dog? I don't care if helmets work, they make you look like a pussy. Why bother riding the bike if you're just gonna look like a bitch doing it? Bro Science isn't about doing what is best for fitness, it's about doing what is best for you, because you are the best. And everyone needs to know it. Now I'm going to beta test some exercises to see which ones you should avoid for your own good.

Hip Machines

I don't even know why I'm here or why I need to be explaining this to you. First off, hip machines are for legs. And not the cooler parts like quads, which is like saying you're the coolest kid at the Renaissance fair. Hip machines train the muscles that help you bear a child. Who cares how important hip abductors and adductors are for building strength? The only point to lifting legs and I mean *the* only point is to make them look bigger so people don't make fun of you when you're forced to wear shorts at the beach. So why are we now worried about leg strength? It's like doing the extra problems in the back of the math book so you can be better at math. What's the fucking point? You ever gonna need to squat 500lbs at your goddamn cubicle during your fuckin' teleconference? What, are you gonna use the quadratic equation to figure out how many beers you need to buy for your bro trip to Canada? No, that's why it has the word "quad" in it. Because "quad" is Latin for useless.

Hip Thrusts

One of the best exercises for building glute strength so you can deadlift more. And I don't mean more often, which is probably more important since you deadlift like once every two months and then hurt yourself because your glutes are too weak. Hip thrusts are also one of the best exercises for looking like a chick having her panties slid off and getting pounded in the mish. So unless you wanna abort your manhood, better pull out, and pull up.

Assisted Pull-ups, or Dips

Time for some word association; my therapist makes me do this. When I hear the word "assisted" I think assisted living. In other words, a bunch of geezers who need help to stay alive. Is this you? Do you need help doing basic things such as moving your own body weight? Okay, old guy from *Up*, text me on your gigantic Jitterbug cell phone when you decide to join the living.

Fixed Barbell Bench

If you want to bench, but you're not strong enough to bench 135 with a barbell, you have two options:

1. Load up the barbell with smaller plates. This is like getting a blow job with a condom on; don't bother unless you're gonna do the real thing.
2. Bench with the fix barbells that only go up to 115lbs max. This is like fingering a fifi . . . with a condom on your fingers. You are not just unfit, you are unfit for society.

Or option 3: Be fucking stronger.

Tricep Kickback

Chicks do this to try to "tone" their flabby underarms. Yeah, these are not bad for getting some tricep detail, but how often do you really do them? You ever get juiced up for a sick set of 20lb kickbacks? Bent over with your ass out and head up, looking like you're jacking off two dudes on either side of you? No way, bro.

Bicep Curl to Shoulder Press

This exercise screams, "I'm new to the gym and I saw a basketball player doing these on an ESPN clip." Doing bicep curls to shoulder press means you're grabbing any weight and just lifting in the first way that comes to mind. You're constantly looking at your own arms, confused, like, "Why am I doing this? Is this right?" You're combining two things that are awesome on their own but suck together . . . like blowback. Blow, awesome. Back, huge. Blowback, cost of doing business.

Buddy Curls

You think this is some sick superbro shit like you and your homie are double-teaming this weight. But really you look like you're slow dancing at eighth-grade homecoming and too shy to just fucking kiss.

There is no point to this, just put the weight on the floor and let him pick it up for his next set, or just come out and be proud that you two ass bang each other.

Shadow Boxing with Weights

This is the same as the guy who practices his golf swing in the office. If you were good at golf or boxing, you wouldn't be doing them against the air.

Anything on the Smith Machine

There is *no* need for this. Using the Smith machine is like wearing a helmet on a stationary bike. You're losing your gains, you're going nowhere, and you look like a fucking narc. Leave the real drugs and the real weight to the cool kids.

You're a Gym Rat now and it's difficult for people to not see you. Hell, you're well on your way to becoming a Monster, so the last thing you want to be seen doing are some beta-boi movements. You are a leader and dozens of beginner lifters watch your every move in the gym. Make sure you're setting them on the path of becoming alpha.

CHAPTER 44

How to Defeat Your Gym Nemesis

It starts out as a normal day. Wake up at noon, shower up, get back into bed, thirty minutes of "just woke up" selfies, six-egg omelet, crush a season of *Friday Night Lights*, some chicken, then boom: gym time. Wait, spend another hour getting your look right, bro. Don't walk out that door looking like a noob. Okay, go time.

You walk into the gym and don't scan in cuz you're like T-Pain in "Bartender." This has been your standard entrance since the Gym Bro stage. The staff may glare at you, but you're not about to change who you are. But this time, something's different—the dude at the front desk stops you. Bro, WTF, do you know who I am? I'm bee-lining it, about to put this gym on the map with today's lift, and you're trynah block my pump? Are you crazy? I keep my cool. Could be some new guy. Shrug off this mishap and don't let it ruin the flow.

But when you enter the weight room, you stop dead in your tracks. Something's off. The room is crowded, and you sense that you're not the only one here. You scan the room. Couple of chicks reading *Cosmo* on the elliptical, some curl bros hoarding the 35s, a lost CrossFitter doing pull-ups. Things seem normal enough. Then . . . you see him:

A guy. A bro. And he's fucking lifting weight. Your weight. Who the fuck is this dude? Does he think he's better than you? Touching your weight on today of all days (arm day)? Not on your watch.

Fuck. This. Guy. This disgrace is officially your gym nemesis.

Listen, anyone who works out as much as you do will eventually find a nemesis. It's just the way life is. Every superhero needs a villain to fuck up. At some point you will meet your Venom . . . except you want to be Venom. Spider-Man is a bitch.

Let me break down what your nemesis looks like. He's the dude who is a similar size to you, similar build, sorta looks like you, probably crushes the same type of pussy as you, and has the same style, but he's def biting yours. You two are competing in the same weight class and he is your direct competition. You have established yourself as the undisputed champ at six feet, 170 pounds, sorta cut, strong on incline dumbbell, and the bro that is in the dungeon every day from 2:00 P.M. to 4:00 P.M. And now this poser is here. In your weight room. He's pretending like he's all minding his own business, but don't doubt for a second that he's trying to take your belt. Not today, Pacquiao.

It's time to go on the offensive. Size him up from a distance.

First, locate something to hide behind. This will be difficult given how fucking huge you are. I recommend stacking a bunch of jump boxes. Good. Now run through your checklist to make sure you aren't giving your nemesis any ill-conceived props. Arms, chest, shoulders: Are mine bigger? Am I stronger? He's about to lift that, it's heavy, what's his form like? Damn, not bad. Still inconclusive, though. Back to his arms, are they bigger? Am I taller? My dick is, for sure.

It is crucial that you find a way to pick apart this douchebag and bring him down so you can get back on top . . . As the famous masstrophysicist and skipper of leg day, Steven Bulking, has proven: Space and time are relative, but pointless. The only thing that matters is mass. And mass is also relative. You are only big if you are bigger than something else that is also big. And as body dysmorphia dictates, you cannot tell how big you are by simply looking at your muscles. You need a side-by-side analysis performed. Luckily, all gyms come equipped with this software: the mirror.

Now that you have completed your analysis, it's time to start moving your workout closer to your nemesis. Don't raise any alarms. The last thing you want is him catching you looking at him and thinking you are 'mirin'.

After executing the side-by-side mirror check, the jury is still out. He could've had better lighting, which means a better pump at the time. There's a 90 percent chance you're bigger than him, and a 10 percent chance he thinks you're gay for him. But joke's on him, the only thing you're gay for is yourself.

You've meandered around the gym trying to imitate your standard workout routine while keeping a close eye on this dude. It seems that he's definitely following you. And it has nothing to do with you inching closer to him and using the same equipment. He wants you dead. Or worse, wants you to be smaller than him. Since the mirrors were obviously ripped from a carnival funhouse and the lighting is clearly skewed in his favor, you need to bring in outside judges. Don't ask for anyone's opinion, just grab your boy and start talking shit about the guy.

Fuck this. You leave this workout feeling like the gym is cheating on you with this impostor. The worst part is, you come back to the Iron Church the next day, and he's there again. Then the next day, same thing. Now you gotta see fucking Reebok every day acting like he's Nike.

Time goes on and tension builds. You hate this guy more than you hate girls who don't give blow jobs. Eventually the gloves come off and you take notice of each other. Probably because you've been working out next to each other for five fucking weeks. You put enough bears on the ice, eventually it's gonna break. What do I mean by this? You can only be near someone for so long before talking about your muscles. At some point, one of you has to brag.

You should expect the conversation to be something like:

You: Yo, I've never done that for biceps, is it good?

Nemesis: Oh, fuck yeah. You're going to get a nasty stretch and it's going to hit—

You (interrupting): I usually do, like, 60s or 70s and really curl it at the top. I mean, it works, as you can see.

Nemesis: Yeah, dude, I can tell. You have huge arms.

Bingo. Just like that, you become bros because being bros with this dude is like being friends with the only person you actually want to be friends with: yourself. When he talks about his biceps, it's like he's talking about your biceps, which he is because the only reason you asked about his biceps was so you could talk about yours, which are bigger. And better. Fuck this guy.

CHAPTER 45

Do You Even Lift?

Okay, hotshot. Just because you actually lift weights or think you might be in shape doesn't mean you're going to get any credit for lifting. You should know by now that getting credit from other lifters or yourself is impossible in this sport. After painstaking years of research in the field, I have created a flowchart to answer the age-old question: Do you even lift?

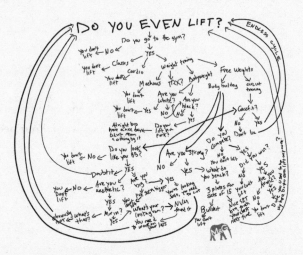

And that proves it. As you can see, no matter what you do, how good you look, no matter how strong you are, even if you're Arnold . . . there's no way around it. You might think you lift, but do you even?

STAGE 6

Monster

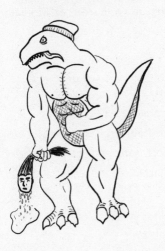

Dude, you're fucking huge. The Gym Rat you once were is terrified of you, and you are terrified of ever going backward. Your need to be bigger than everyone has led you to experiment with "extracurriculars" and other risky methods scored from the fanny packs of shady locker room trolls. This doesn't worry you one bit. Your boy just got out of med school and gives you under-the-table checkups every week to make sure you're juicing correctly. People are trying to tell you that this "career" you've chosen is short term, but you literally cannot hear them because they're too small to matter.

Chicks? What chicks? You're not interested in wasting your time with women when you could be shoveling nutrients into your mouth, walking around the gym scaring people out of the squat rack, or sleeping. Doesn't matter anyway, cuz girls look at you and think you have a problem. *Good*. Because you do. It's called "I can still fit through doorways."

At this point the gym is the only thing you do, the only thing you care about, and the only thing you're good at. You've been doing it for so long that you've forgotten what it's like to be a human . . . or look like one. Because you're not one. You're a Monster. Both physically and emotionally.

CHAPTER 46

Pros and Cons of Taking Steroids

Decision time. You've been lifting for a few years now, and you've hit some plateaus. You're starting to catch on that a lot of lifters are "supplementing their income." Your boys that you thought were natty all this time, well, it turns out they've been juicin' since Capri Sun.

Your reality has shifted. You're at a crossroads: To the left, you got twenty miles to a weekend in Vegas and your life savings in your pocket. You're gonna hit highs you will never hit anywhere else. And to the right, you got the unpaved cross-country dirt road to that house with a family and a sustainable life. What's more important? Thought so.

So for those Monsters out there that are on the fence about supplementing their income, allow the Brofessor to break down the pros and cons of taking steroids.

The Pros

MAD GAINS

No-fucking-brainer. This is what you're here for, isn't it? This is grabbing your controller and hitting Triangle, R2, Left, L1, X, Right,

Triangle, Down, Square, L1, L1, L1. Boom. Unlimited guns, unlimited ammo. I mean, ya still gotta play the game, but once you enter the code you're never gonna play again without it.

YOU GET STRONGER

It's not about how much you can lift, it's about how much you look like you can lift, but it helps if you can lift a lot, too. If gains are Jordan, then strength is Pippen. Jordan could probably do it by himself, but Pippen did his part. But I'll tell ya one thing: I never had a fuckin' Pippen poster hanging on my wall.

CUTS AND VEINS

You will finally achieve that "my skin looks like a leaf" look. Your body fat will be nonexistent and terrified of ever returning. Where you once had skin, you'll now have veins; where you once had veins, you'll now have more veins. Your bicep vein alone is going to look like an aerial shot of the Mississippi splitting off into a shitload of other huge rivers.

THERE WILL BE ZERO DOUBT THAT YOU LIFT

Your muscles are so dense they look like a tight bag of rocks. No one will ever question your dedication to the Iron Church. Swolemates at the gym will ask you to officiate at their wedding. You'll decline, because you'll be in the gym.

FAST RECOVERY

You're racing NASCAR, and you never need to make a pit stop. All you do is win.

INCREASED LIBIDO

Your sex drive is a monster truck. It will go anywhere and crush anything.

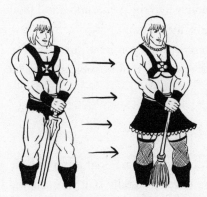

Juicing is a double-edged sword. One edge is super sharp and can slice through Wolverine's claws. The other edge is kind of dull, a little round, and not really going to turn any heads with its slicing ability. But hey, fair is fair. And now that we've explored the benefits of juicing, let's see what the other side has to offer.

Cons

STEROIDS FUCK WITH YOUR NATURAL TESTOSTERONE

When you're on, you're golden . . . but when you get off, you start growing bitch tits, and your dick stops working. Overnight, you go from he-man to wo-man.

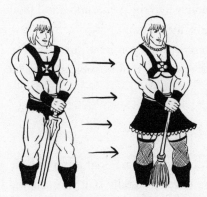

Your life is changing in front of your very eyes and it's all your fault. Worst of all, you know the reason why this is happening is in the fanny pack of that sketchy dude posted outside the gym. Such a simple solution, right there in front of you. But you took the high road, bro. Enjoy it.

EMOTIONAL INSTABILITY

On the outside you look rock solid. But on the inside you're Michael J. Fox on a trampoline playing Jenga against an actual time bomb. Like, the other day I saw my boy jump out of his car at an intersection and threaten a traffic light with a knife because his favorite color is blue. Then later that day I walked in on him sitting alone in the dark bawling his eyes out to the beginning of *Titanic*. Not a good look, bro. I mean, I've cried to *Titanic* before, except the tears came out of my dick.

JUICE IS EXPENSIVE

Okay, maybe you got no problem investing five, ten, fifteen, twenty years of your life for some right-now fucking gains, duh. But now you also gotta dip into your 401(k) to fund this meat market. You already invest all your money into the gym, supps, and food . . . in that order. You see your bank account and put some serious thought into quitting this new lifestyle, then you look in the mirror a week later and immediately pick up every shift possible at your job. It's time to put in work.

NEEDLES

It's not like pounding down some Gnar Pump, which tastes like fuckin' house music. You have to literally stab yourself and inject chemicals into your blood. As cool as this sounds, it's fuckin' dark, bro.

HAVING TO EXPLAIN TO YOUR DOCTOR FOR THE MILLIONTH TIME THAT IT'S COOL

He spent twelve years studying the body; you spent twelve months building the body. You don't need to listen to his bullshit science for regular people, cuz I'm an animal and last I checked you're not a vet. So beat it, Dr. Islittle.

AND HERE ARE FEW "FACTS" ABOUT THE "NEGATIVES" OF STEROID USE THAT I PRINTED OUT FROM MEDICALJOURNAL.COM

Steroids

- enlarge your organs
- raise blood pressure
- increase chances of heart attack over time
- make you hairy
- mess up your reproductive system
- cause liver damage
- raise cholesterol
- cause acne
- cause sterilization
- lead to cardiovascular problems
- cause kidney problems
- promote excessive sweating
- increase risk of HIV and Hep B and C from needles
- increase the risk of psychosis

- cause aching joints
- cause insomnia
- lead to depression

Yada, yada, yada. At the end of the day, it's your choice, just like it was your choice to become the Monster that you are. Point is, no one's gonna stop you because no one can stop you.

CHAPTER 47

People You Hate at the Gym

The gym is filled with people you hate. Some people you hate because you're a hater and everyone is taking up your space, some you hate because even their parents hate them, but others you hate because they are fucking with your gains. Aka gain rapists. These are the worst people in the gym. Here's the rundown of some of the worst offenders.

The Guy Who Wants You to Work Out Faster

Fuck this old crab. He ain't working in for shit. This is always some old dude who asks how many you got left on set one and is always unhappy with the answer. He looks at you all confused and irritated, acting like you didn't give up your subway seat to a pregnant lady that just boarded. Then he lingers around the entire time giving you the stink eye while you're cruising Instagram in between sets. Fuck off, Dumbledore, I'm not trying to catch your scabies from Ellis Island. He just wants you to work out faster cuz he's gonna die soon.

The Guy Who Wants to Work In Even Though It's Gonna Really Complicate the Exercise

You're doing squats, and this guy comes over asking to work in. Then, after you agree, he springs it on you that he's gonna be doing bench with the safeties up. Then he asks you to help strip the weight and rearrange everything. This is like that friend who will ask you for a favor, but doesn't tell you what it is until after you reply yes. And now you're stuck being the godfather of his kid because it's too late to ignore his text. Which is fine until your friend kicks the bucket and then you're stuck looking out for his loser kid who is def gonna grow up to masturbate to dragons and shit. That's on you now.

The Guy Who Puts the Weights Back in the Wrong Spot

This guy must have dropped out of school, cuz he never learned how to count by five or match shapes. Now, thanks to Count von Count, I have to grab one of the 90s from the top shelf of the rack and the other 90 from the opposite end, both equally far from my bench and the numbered slot that says "90lbs" but has 15lb DBs in it. I don't want to be digging through six layers of 5s, 10s, and 25s, to get to the 45 like I'm unearthing a rubber from my sock drawer at 4:00 A.M.

The Guy Who Works Out in Front of Your Mirror Space

If there wasn't a mirror, there would be a chance you might not have noticed me working out behind you. But I know you can see me working out behind you. You know how I know this? Because you're standing in front of a fucking mirror. And before your selfish ass got in the way, I could see me, too, and so could everyone else. I could see my pump, my glory, and my future. And now all I can see is your back fat and the reason your wife left you two years ago.

The Guy Who Works Right off the Rack

This is the dude who goes to Whole Foods and eats all the fucking produce off the shelf acting like he's checking for freshness like it's his personal fucking garden. Nah, it's cool, I don't need any of the grapes that you mauled with your inconsiderate gypsy fingers. I'll just stand here and wait for more to grow.

The Guy Who Works Out Super Close to You

You're mid-set benching 100lb DBs over your face, and this dude thinks it's a good time to sit next to you and flap around some seated lateral raises. This guy was never taught the concept of personal space. After he's done with his set, you can bet he's gonna stare at you in the mirror and scare away all your gains. Now I know how chicks feel.

Anyone Doing CrossFit

I don't want to be inhaling your fucking chalk dust while I'm mid-set just so you can have enough grip to hold onto the pull-up bar that you're violently swinging from while your friend is busy giving himself scoliosis with the barbell I've been waiting for since I got here. You really need all that equipment to make zero gains? This is the dude that rocks True Religion jeans, a vest, and a fedora to the bar just to get zero pussy.

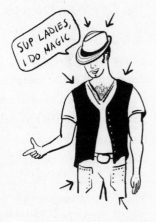

Who are you trying to fool, bro? I can literally see your virginity.

The Guy Who Does the Tricep Dips on Two Benches

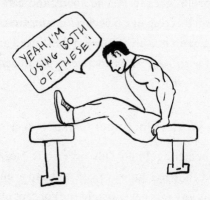

Benches in the gym are like outlets in airports; people kill for that shit. Doing tricep dips on two benches is like claiming two beds at a party just so you can push 'em together and sleep in the crack.

The Guy Who Does Cable Swings in the Middle of the Cable Cross

You're trying to hit tricep push-down, but Arnold Palmer is standing dead center in the cable cross, swinging the cables like shaving a couple of strokes off his golf game is gonna get his dick to work again. And now he's gotta turn around and hit his other side. He's using one cable, but taking up both sides for twice as long. Give it a rest, the only sand trap you haven't been in lately is your wife's vag.

The Guy Who Snipes Your Setup and Completely Rearranges It by the Time You're Back from the Water Fountain

This guy's the worst. I leave for fifteen seconds, then this dude, probably named Franco, rolls up and ignores the fact that I left all my shit on the bench and the weight on the bar. This, coincidentally, is the same dude who's always trying to convince your chick to break up with you every time you're not around, saying he's got tickets to Sam Smith and that he knows she deserves to be treated better. Piss off, Jafar. You don't know me. I leave for fifteen seconds and you think you can fuck with my setup? This ain't a game! Talk to my chick all you want, but don't fuck with my setup!

There will always be people you hate at the gym, but if you haven't noticed, the bigger you've gotten the less these people annoy you because it's getting harder for you to see them and easier for them to see you. These herbs immediately take notice of you and choose to spectate from afar rather than even think about doing their workout anywhere near you. There are countless types of annoying people bringing shame to the Iron Church. If you have any offenders at your gym, immediately submit a report to your local authorities. See something, say something. #Brofficer #SwolePatrol #MakeAmericaSwoleAgain.

CHAPTER 48

How to Declare War on New Year's Resolutioners

The gym is the worst in January. Not because it's crowded—you love when the gym is crowded. Crowds equal witnesses, witnesses equal attention, and as we know, attention is the primary source of muscle growth.

No, the reason you hate the gym in January is because the gym is *your* thing. You've been doing it longer and better than anyone on earth. In fact, right after gravity was invented by Bisaac Newton, you said fuck gravity and invented antigravity, which later became known as lifting as soon as you set foot in the gym. Just because the fucking date's changed, everyone thinks they can do your thing. Lemme tell you something: Lifting isn't just your thing, it's your only thing, and if everyone starts doing your one thing then you'll have no thing, and therefore you will become nothing. So it's time to declare war on these resolutioners and take action before these noobs take your gains.

Start a Revolution

Broadcast your frustration on social media. This shows the world that you aren't a resolutioner. The year might be new, but this shit ain't.

You've been going to the gym since *the* new year, like, the first one. Year one. BC! Here are some ways to take it to social media:

> Post an angry status about hating resolutioners. Remember, they aren't people with goals trying to better themselves, they are developing-world refugees trying to take all our jobs; by jobs I mean gains.

> Share articles written by journalists on why resolutioners are the worst. These are extremely insightful works of literature.

> Instagram an accurate meme showing how accurately crowded the gym is after New Year's. Literally make the resolutioners get in the fucking picture.

Instill Fear into Your Enemy

You can achieve this by doing a lot of huffing and puffing. Make your anger known . . . and seen, and heard publicly by everyone with eyes or ears, or just create a general sense of negative energy.

Going to the gym in January is like being stuck in traffic. You aren't just another car adding to the problem, you are the *only* car and all the others are the problem. You are the only one with a right to be mad, because you run this place. Duh.

Build Your Army

Pull people aside and explain to them how crowded the gym is. You want to separate yourself from the resolutioners. If you don't actively complain to people about other people, you might be mistaken for one of them.

Claim Your Territory

Set up camp by bringing more gear than you normally do and scattering it around your equipment. Now plant your flag by maxing out set one, so everyone knows where to find America. Don't mess with a superpower.

With all this greatness going down, you need to protect your house. Keep your equipment locked down during rest periods. I usually pile on a bunch of dumbbells over whatever I'm using that are too heavy for normal people to lift.

Go to War

Since it's impossible to literally tell everyone in the gym that you've been coming here first, lift like your life depends on it, so it's impossible for them not to know. Go to war with the fucking weight, and win. If you need to come into the gym in full army gear with face paint like you just got back from Vietnam, then you do it. Plus, that's a good look either way. #ForrestPump.

—◖———◗—

Bro, I know how painful January can be for you. It will take every ounce of patience you have, which isn't much cuz of the juice. But you will make it through the toughest time of year because you always do. You are a Monster. It's clear to you and to everyone else that you run the gym and you will be putting up weight when the New Year's resolutioners arrive and long after they leave.

CHAPTER 49

How to Bring a Beginner to the Gym

Why would anyone go through the hassle of bringing a beginner to the gym? For the same reason anyone goes through the hassle of bringing a kid into the world: You're in your late twenties, you've been out of college for a few years, you have a boring job, and you have nothing interesting left to offer to the world, so you need something in your life to get those Facebook likes rolling in again. And, like bringing up a kid, raising a gym newbie is the perfect way to force your values onto someone else; you can end up with the perfect gym buddy. You're already a father figure to so many gym bros, but it might be time to adopt a brotégé.

You've been hitting up the same gym since you started lifting. Those mirrors have seen you through every stage of your lifting evolution, while others have come and gone. You take pride in knowing that the knurling on the barbells has given you more blisters than anyone who's run through your mecca. You're the Godfather, the Brofessor of your gym. When you're on the bench repping 315 to warm up, a line forms waiting to ask for your advice. At this point you're basically the owner, even though you still pay full price for your yearly membership. Something is missing, though. You are more obsessed with yourself than ever, but you want to give back. The other day, daycare chick asked you if you have any kids. What the fuck was she thinking with a question like that? But, it got you thinking that maybe you are ready to bring another human into your world. So instead of rolling the dice by sexing up another 'roided-out lifter chick, you bring in a beginner. A soft, malleable bag of feathers. Someone to look up to you. Someone to mold into a hard, chiseled back of rocks. Your brotégé.

This is the biggest step you've taken in your life, so don't fuck it up. Sure, your brotégé is going to have an actual mother and father, but you're the one turning him into a well-rounded, self-obsessed muscle warrior. Here's how to make sure your brotégé passes his classes, then goes on to skip college and become a brofessor, just like you.

The First Gym Session

You're at the gym waiting for the noob to show up for more than an hour. He's not late . . . you just never left. When he finally shows up, you actually consider bailing on him, moving to another city, and switching your gym membership. You expected him to have zero gym style, but you weren't ready for this. He's wearing actual gym clothes.

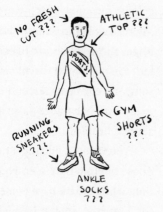

This fucking guy; dressed like he's going to work out, like he's going to exercise. Hey, Jane Fonda, we're going to the gym, not an eighties theme party. Where's your swag? This is a gym—it's about looking fresh, not looking fresh off the boat.

> **BRO TIP:** Always carry an emergency swag pack. The swag pack consists of emergency backup gym gear you always have at the ready. You never know when you'll need to grab a quick pump and you gotta look fresh, so you're always prepared. In this case, your brotégé needs the swag more than you.

Would you let your kid out of the house looking like an orphan? Didn't think so. You can't let people think you accept another human looking like a noob under your jurisdiction. You have a reputation to protect. Bless him with your swag pack, aka some of your spare dirty clothes, and make him go change. Even though everything is three sizes too big for him, he'll be thanking you one day . . . the day that they're too small.

Now that he is all dressed for school, it's time to graduate him with a degree in Bro Science. The first class is a pass/fail: Intro to Pre-Workout. It's pass the scoop and fail at nothing.

Your noob's fight or flight instinct will kick in, and he's going to stupidly ask if it's okay to take pre-workout. Now's your chance to flex your knowledge, aka your biceps, and remind him who's teaching the class . . . and fucking the TA on the side.

Noob: Is this safe?

Dom Flexes: You see this? Anymore questions?

Noob: Yes, a lot actually.

Now that your brotégé bossed up and chugged his delicious pre-workout for the first time, it's time to head into the dojo. When entering the weight room, be sure to walk at least ten paces ahead of him. You want there to be

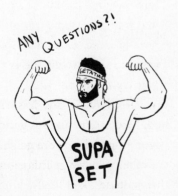

zero confusion about who the leader is here. The captain doesn't sit in fucking coach, he flies the goddamn plane, behind a barricaded door. These pigeons haven't earned their wings yet.

Explaining Exercises

Teaching isn't about showing people what they need to know; it's about showing people how much you already know. When explaining an exercise to a beginner, you get to lift, show off your muscles, and talk about them, all at the same time. It's like scoring a touchdown while calling the play-by-play for your own highlight reel.

Choosing weight for a beginner sucks. They have no idea how much they can lift, so it's all in your hands. My advice is don't pick a weight that is appropriate for a beginner to lift, pick a weight that is appropriate for you to look at. I'm not going to be stacking 45s outside these 25s like some classless troglodyte. You're starting with 45s whether you like it or not, or can do it or not. Not my problem.

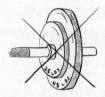

Spotting

Watching a beginner try to lift for the first time is like watching a baby whale try to unbeach itself. There's a lot of wiggling and oceanic weeping. It's sad, really. You don't understand how a human can't get their body to do something so basic and instinctual. The key to teaching a beginner proper form is to shout names of body parts and technical cues they've never heard before, then uncomfortably smack and poke their muscles, and finally jump in and finish their set for them. Actions speak louder than words, even though I'm fucking shouting.

Post-Workout

Thank god that's over. You did good, though. You completed a selfless act that was definitely seen by everyone in the gym. Well, really that lift session wasn't so bad. You got to lift your normal body part and superset it with his entire workout and now your pump is legendary. Hand the kid his first protein shake, recap the workout, and talk about how sore he is going to be.

Being a brofessor is a tough gig, but there are benefits to it. You take great satisfaction in flexing your knowledge and showing off your pump. You were somebody again for ninety minutes, but now all that is left is for your pump to fade and you to realize you don't want this kind of responsibility. You popped out the kid, you got the attention you needed, but now you're stuck raising him. Yet, you feel gratified, like you contributed to something bigger than yourself. Wait, that's bullshit. That noob ain't bigger than you!

CHAPTER 50

Meathead Goals

In case you haven't noticed, lifting is all about setting up impossible goals, and then becoming bigger than them. You saw each goal paraded in front of you from the day you set foot in the gym. That dude putting up 135 on bench—goal. The homie shoulder pressing 80s—next goal. Those meat titans deadlifting five plates—goal. Overcoming your next plateau hinges on setting up your muscle brain to lift more weight. Simple as that. The gym is your world and you need to be the leader of it. So, here are a few goals to keep yourself at the center of the *you*niverse.

Pursue Your Dreams

Quit your job and finally become a personal trainer, because you like to lift and you're an expert at science and muscles and things and shit. At first, it'll feel good to know that you've established yourself enough to give people lifting advice and get paid for it. But, eventually, you will realize you hate personal training, because you only care about your own gains, so you start your lucrative in-house business selling Herbalife supplements on your sick social media network. They don't teach that in business school; they don't teach that *any*where. You also sell steroids! If you, like, need them, and shit. Don't tell anyone, though.

Get a New Hobby That Doesn't Involve Yourself

Photography is a good place to start. And by photography, I mean become a professional selfie taker. What good is overcoming your goal if you're not documenting it, bro? In the old days lifters used to carry around these things called a pen and paper. They would actually record in written form every lift completed, analyze them, and assess how close they were to completing their goal. You can still view their findings inside caves and museums across the world. Today, all you do is take several selfies every chance you get. You are your favorite muse anyway, and your only muse, so why not take it to the next level. Throw a couple #Herbalife hashies in there, push your pics to the 'gram, and you're in the green.

Start Reading

Reading is great for making those sick brain gains. It's a great way to learn new things and discover new words. It may be too difficult to locate some reading material, so a great place to start is supplement labels. There are tons of words on there that no one has discovered. You will not only become great at dishing out generic lifting tips to randoms at the gym, but you can sling a bunch of real science out there, too. You're a double threat.

Take Risks

Go for that one-rep-max bench you've been lying to yourself about for years. Don't even warm up. You can do it. Most people take time to break through to their next goal; not you. You had all of last year to warm up. Just go for it and don't bother with a spot either; it's not self-improvement if you can't do it yourself. As they say, the biggest risk is not taking one; the risk of course being pre-workout and other substances.

Actually Take a Cycle Off Pre-Workout

Face it, you've probably been taking pre-workout nonstop for years, and including a time bomb of health concerns, you've probably also built up a tolerance that requires you to take six scoops and stack it with a 9-volt battery in order to feel a slight buzz. So maybe it's time to take a week off, like you've been telling yourself you should, like the label has urged you to, and like your bloodwork has indicated.

Rinse Your Protein Shaker After Using It

You probably have about six or seven shaker cups that you've accumulated from bodybuilding orders. All of which are currently sitting in the sink, sealed with your dirty last sip of protein sitting at the bottom, which has now developed this Greek-yogurt-type film and a layer of congealed bacteria.

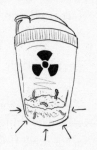

This is the worst smell on earth and also how the world will end. It takes five seconds to rinse your cup and save humanity. Commit to doing this on the reg.

Lend a Helping Hand

This year and every year after, and before, may be all about improving yourself, but try to take a moment to help out the little guys. If you see a smaller being struggling to curl his weight, or lifting with incorrect form, just calmly walk over, grab the weight out of his hand, and lift his weight for him. Actions speak louder than words.

Your entire life people around you have told you to set goals. Goals for sports you may have played, goals for school, goals for getting a job, etc., etc. You never wanted to, and I don't blame you, because you knew there was something else out there for you. A driving force that would make you want to set goals for yourself. Something you could be great at. Well, you fucking found it, bro. It's there, see it? Look harder. Ah, now you see. He's staring back at you in the mirror, and no matter what size he is, he could be bigger, stare back. Good. Now go crush your next PR.

STAGE 7

Freak Beast

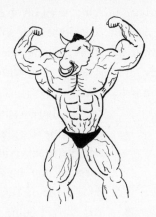

I'm going to be honest with you guys. You may not be able to tell by looking at me, but I have not yet reached the Freak Beast stage. The Freak Beast stage is reserved for the go-hards; the fucking Navy SEALs of the gym who saw their futures the first time they looked at a mirror. You don't encounter a Freak Beast every day. Shit, you're lucky if your gym even has one. These guys are the Olympians. They make Conan the Barbarian look like a starving immigrant fresh off the boat at Ellis Island.

At this point, if you have reached this elite level, you have competed, probably been pro at some point, and are now over it. You have a supplement sponsor, a few half-page ads in *Muscle & Fitness*, and you carry a fucking cooler everywhere full of eight premade meals, aka your lunchbox. You have defied the human form and pushed past so many plateaus you basically conquered Everest five times over. When you have a dinner party, Zeus comes down from the sky and you still out-eat the guy. The only reason a statue isn't made of you is because you'd be bigger than it the next day. You haven't spoken an actual word in over a year because you haven't had a need to. The world knows everything they need to know about you just by looking at you. You actually outgrew having to explain yourself.

Fitness trends? Man, you're not even involved with that shit. You are the trend. Every new lift you add to your split and every piece of gym tech added to your wardrobe becomes the whisper throughout the gym, immediately hits Instagram and eventually the world. And by that point you're on to the next.

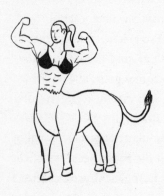

You have a successful Instagram fit profile, make a sizable income off "online" personal training, and are without question the biggest, most shredded dude around. You are Animal Planet. You started going to a vet instead of a doctor two years ago and the girls you used to bang are no longer attracted to you because you are no longer attracted to them. You are now attracted to weird centaur-looking women.

You stopped lifting for chicks a long time ago, cuz the only people who are really gonna care about your veins, and cuts, or how swole your rear delts are are dudes. Your interests, passion, and entire life revolve around the male body. No homo, though. Dudes that pass you on the street have to snap a pic and send it to their crew. You are inspiration in human form.

So when it comes to Bro Science, there ain't nothing you don't know already. You are Bro Science to the nth degree. I salute and thank you for your service.

CONCLUSION

Wow, I never thought I'd say this, but I'm at a loss for words. You have officially completed the first and only book you need to read. Congratulations. You are a learned student of Bro Science and are hereby approved to spread the knowledge to those around you, even if they aren't asking for it. With great knowledge comes great responsibility. Other Bro Scientists to have walked this earth include Stephen Bulking, Swolbroham Lincoln, and Mahatma Gaindhi. You are now a member of the biggest squad known to man.

Most important is that you never lose sight of the journey. When you look in the mirror for ninety minutes each morning, take one of those minutes (max) to remember how you looked a year ago. Or a day ago. Actually, you were definitely a little bigger last year. You caught strep a couple of months ago and haven't recovered yet. But you're more shredded this year. You should actually weigh yourself . . .

Where was I . . . wait, you weigh 220 now? Holy shit, bro.

Think back to when you started reading *The Swoly Bible* and how each page was a piece of your history. You started lifting for a reason, a dream of being big. You definitely made some rookie mistakes along the way, but luckily you had a brofessor to show you the light. Now, you spend so much time in the gym that it's actually your home. You put the front desk guy down as your emergency contact and literally have the gym's address as your "home" shortcut in Google Maps.

Be proud, bro. You woke up one day, looked in the mirror, and made a fucking change. No one but *you* put the work in. So whether you are still in the Gym Bro stage (jealous), graduated to Gym Rat, or went the distance all the way to Freak Beast, you will always be a lifter. It's a small circle you belong to, mostly because everyone in it is so fucking huge, and there's no other circle worth being in.

On behalf of the Bro Scientists worldwide, keep entering the Iron Throne like you are (seven days a week) and getting those gains. If you ever find yourself lost out there, suddenly with a kettlebell in your hand, running outside, or being dragged to some class by a so-called friend, just refer to the Ten Commandments of Bro Science to find your way back to the dumbbells.

The Ten Commandments of Bro Science

1. The day you started lifting was the day you became forever small because you will never be as big as you want to be.
2. It's not about how much you can lift, it's about how much it looks like you can lift.
3. Fitness is 98 percent lighting, the other 2 percent is the sun effect on Instagram.
4. Bench like your life depends on it, because it does.
5. Cardio: running through hoes, swimming in pussy, and cycling pre-workout.
6. Never skip leg day, unless you really need a bicep pump.
7. You *always* need a bicep pump.
8. Thou shalt covet these gains.
9. It is better to be seen as a douchebag than to not be seen at all.
10. Live large, die large, leave a giant coffin.

BRONUS

100 Ways to Say "Jacked"

1. Jacked
2. Ripped
3. Diesel
4. Yolked
5. Buff
6. Swol
7. Brolic
8. Peeled
9. Cut
10. Hard body
11. Juggernaut
12. Minced
13. Beast mode
14. Juiced
15. Cornfed
16. Full housed
17. Swolberham Lincoln
18. Backrocked Obama
19. Ivan Drago
20. USDA buck steak
21. Shredded cheddar
22. Rock swol
23. Torque thunder
24. Bee stung
25. Dee-zel Washington
26. Ox diesel
27. Bull fucked
28. Thunder beast
29. Kilimanjaro
30. Diesel rocket
31. Eiffel power
32. Dikembe Mujumbo
33. Massachussettes
34. Optimus prime
35. Zeus laser
36. Berlin wall
37. Duplex double housed
38. Jupiter tank

39. Colossus
40. Meat titan
41. Campbell's chunky souped
42. Pump dragon
43. Bonecut
44. Diamond cuts
45. Muscle barn
46. Django Unchained
47. 50 shades of gains
48. Muscle bear
49. Double meat
50. Whopper senior
51. Tyrannosaurus flex
52. Poseidon
53. Jesus lean
54. Gandhi cut
55. Swolnight Shyamalan
56. Apollo 45s
57. Juice rifle
58. Radio City Muscle Hall
59. Dial toned
60. World War III
61. Jerry Stackhoused
62. Museum of Muscle History
63. Scruff McBuff
64. Treasure chested
65. Tri sexual
66. Razor sharp
67. Jacked4d
68. Meat sauced
69. Pump nectar
70. Shock blitzed
71. Beef champion
72. Funkmaster Flex
73. Big town straight swol
74. Gaston
75. Thick neck trap housed
76. Armed and dangerous
77. Hotter than the sand, bigger than the ocean
78. Juice box
79. Truck house
80. Paul Bunyon
81. 6pac
82. Wide-armed thunder compound
83. A1 Steak Sauced
84. Armed swoldier
85. Muscles egg and cheese
86. Mufasa
87. Veincity
88. Baconator
89. Stonebreaker
90. Double jacked triple stacked
91. Fleetwood Mac Daddy
92. Donkey brolic
93. Pump jockey
94. Muscle taxi
95. Genetic beast lobster
96. Real-time cage dragon
97. Muscle-grinding cash badger
98. Blood factory
99. Cock diesel
100. Cash rock thunder mammal

ACKNOWLEDGMENTS

Big up to my Dom Squad, aka all my fans who helped make this illiterate gym rat into a published author gym rat.

Other acknowledgments include: Dom Mazzetti, the Brofessor, Domald Pump, Dom Mazzerratti, Dom D to the O M, Dom O. Mazzetti (the O is for O-wesome), D-Train, Dom "Keep It Open" Mazzetti, me. Your boi. The dude. Numero Uno. Bye, haterz.